VERONICA PEARSON

Mental Health Care in China

State Policies, Professional Services and
Family Responsibilities

GASKELL

© The Royal College of Psychiatrists 1995

Gaskell is an imprint of the Royal College of Psychiatrists,
17 Belgrave Square, London SW1X 8PG

All rights reserved. No part of this book may be reprinted or
reproduced or utilised in any form or by any electronic,
mechanical, or other means, now known or hereafter invented,
including photocopying and recording, or in any information
storage or retrieval system, without permission in writing from the
publishers.

British Library Cataloguing-in-Publication Data
A catalogue record for this book is available from
the British Library.

ISBN 0-902241-74-5

Distributed in North America
by American Psychiatric Press, Inc.
ISBN 0-88048-639-2

The views presented in this book do not necessarily reflect those
of the Royal College of Psychiatrists, and the publishers are not
responsible for any error of omission or fact.

The Royal College of Psychiatrists is a registered charity (no.228636).

Contents

iv

For Felicity, Michael, Nicholas and Eleanor

Acknowledgements

An enterprise of this nature is never the result of just one person's effort. While I am not necessarily in a position to repay the debts I have accrued, I can at least acknowledge them. Much of the research on which this book is based was made possible with grants from two sources: the Keswick Foundation of Hong Kong (a John Keswick scholarship) and the University of Hong Kong's Research and Conference Grants Committee. The work would not have been possible without their support.

I was very fortunate to have the help of a number of hardworking and efficient research assistants at different times: Tim Chan, Edith Chang, Roger Kwan, May Tam, and Mandy Yiu. Very special thanks go to Rose Yu, who accompanied me on virtually all my trips to the Municipal Hospital (Chapter 5) over a period of five years. Her patience, good humour (under sometimes rather trying circumstances) and wisdom were remarkable and my debt to her is considerable.

Various colleagues and friends have provided assistance and support, among whom I would particularly like to mention Ms Lindsay Barker, Dr Cecilia Chan, Professor Nelson Chow, Dr Michael Phillips, and Dr Linda Wong. The draft manuscript benefited from the careful reading and insightful comments of Ms Marlys Bueber, Mr John Carpenter, Ms Sarah Howroyd, Dr Stewart MacPherson and Dr Liz McLean.

I would also like to acknowledge the help and hospitality from the many psychiatrists in China with whom I have worked over the years and from whom I have learned much. My hope is that the opening up that China has experienced over the last fifteen years will continue, and that the barriers to the exchange of ideas between Chinese psychiatrists and those from Western countries will continue to dissolve.

Finally, my thanks are due to Professor Kathleen Jones whose knowledge, and boundless enthusiasm, have been available to me since the inception of this project.

Introduction

To suffer from severe mental illness in any society is a potential tragedy, often compounded by stigma and a sense of shame for both patients and their families. In China the position is no different from that in other countries. In some ways it is worse, because of the Chinese government's unwillingness to be open about the situation of people with a mental illness (Kleinman, 1986). Mental illness is regarded as not only shameful for the family but also for the whole country. This level of prejudice is reflected in the health declaration that foreign visitors must complete on entering China. Psychosis is bracketed with leprosy and AIDS (two of the most feared diseases in Asia) as the three specifically named illnesses about which foreigners are questioned.

This official attitude of secrecy towards mental illness means that there is little reliable information available about what goes on in Chinese psychiatric hospitals, despite the numerous reports by Western observers that are based on brief visits to Chinese psychiatric facilities. Some of these reports are politically influenced. Other observers may lack sufficient background knowledge of the Chinese situation and are able to do little more than report what they have seen and been told.

Clearly, there is a need for empirical studies that will give some sense of the realities of psychiatric care in China, although these must necessarily be limited in scope. Anyone who wishes to study aspects of life in China quickly becomes aware of the vastness and diversity of the country. At the time of my first visit to a Chinese psychiatric hospital (the Shanghai Number One, in 1983) there seemed little hope of being able to do research because of the very restrictive attitude of the Chinese authorities towards contact with outsiders. As the 1980s progressed, however, the effects of China's 'open door' policy towards the outside world became

1

apparent. There was a positive desire to learn more about Western ideas, not just in the area of business and investment but in science, technology and medicine. Opportunities for research in the field of mental illness became available. My professional and research activities have always been largely concerned with the care of people with a mental illness and so it seemed natural, when living and working in Hong Kong, to extend this focus to China.

Over the years I have visited at least 16 different psychiatric hospitals in China, varying from the premier hospitals in Beijing and Shanghai to small county level hospitals in Shandong and Sichuan. Some of these visits have been extensive enough to permit me to undertake research, for instance in Hubei province and Beijing, as well as substantial teaching programmes. Since 1992, I have presented papers at five conferences within China on psychiatric care and in 1991 I was appointed adviser to the Ministry of Civil Affairs' National Training Centre for Mental Health Workers.

Officially, the population of China is 1.16 billion people, constituting about one-quarter of the human race. Although to an outsider the Chinese people appear homogeneous, there are in fact many divisions. There are differences between the rural and urban populations, between coastal and interior provinces and between the minority peoples and the dominant Han Chinese. Even among the latter, there are many dialect groups and there is a perception of separateness between people from the various parts of China. The sheer size of the country means that any empirical work must take account of this variability. In the past, a strong centralised administration imposed a degree of uniformity. However, with the pursuit of a more open economy since 1978, it has proved increasingly difficult for the national government to impose its will on the provinces and large cities.

It is difficult, if not impossible, for research workers in the field of social policy to avoid being influenced by their own attitudes, both in their choice of topic and the way they select and interpret data. It is necessary therefore for the reader to know what these attitudes are and how they were formed.

My viewpoint is that major mental illness, particularly schizophrenia, is very often a tragedy for both patients and their families. It is destructive of lives and generates fear rather than sympathy in others. Despite the potential resources available to help and support patients and relatives, not enough is done to alleviate the burden that they carry.

I have no personal doubt that schizophrenia exists and that it is an illness, although the aetiology is complex and imperfectly understood. In China I have interviewed patient after patient, all exhibiting symptoms of acute psychotic disorder that are immediately recognisable. Families have described to me a similar range of problems in coping with someone with this disorder as those I have come across in my social work practice in the United Kingdom. They receive little support from either medical or social services, and neighbours and workmates are frequently unhelpful or even hostile. Difficulties regarding accommodation, work, finances and marriage also loom large in their experience.

At present, there is a deep division between those who support the exclusively medical view of mental illness, and those who support the social view, that much or all of what is classified as 'mental illness' is concerned with problems in human relationships, and that medical labels are stigmatising. My view, that both sides in this debate would benefit from a greater understanding and respect for the other viewpoint, is based on the wholly practical grounds that only through the application of understanding and insights gained from both social science and medicine can we offer an effective service to users.

Much of what follows is concerned with problems associated with schizophrenia. This is partly due to personal experience of people with this chronic and disabling condition, but there are other reasons. First, the issue of the reliability and frequency of the diagnosis of depression and manic depression in China is very controversial (Kleinman, 1986; Young & Xiao, 1993), while schizophrenia is generally accepted to occur in all societies. (Sartorius *et al*, 1986; Jablensky, 1988). In addition, schizophrenia is easier to identify than other forms of mental illness, and comparisons with the West tend to be more reliable.

Second, schizophrenia is seen by the Chinese themselves as the major problem facing psychiatrists and psychiatric services. Yan *et al* (1980) and Yan & Xiang (1984) confirm that over 80% of psychiatric patients are given this diagnosis. Kleinman & Lin (1981, p.139) point out that:

"With their practical concern for providing adequate care to the severely ill and minimising the impact of mental illness on community productivity and social order, the Chinese psychiatrists have undoubtedly been more interested in schizophrenia than in other kinds of psychiatric affliction."

Third, more than any other psychiatric illness, schizophrenia has profound consequences for sufferers and their families. The chronic, debilitating nature of the disease, its potential to disrupt social relationships and the limitations of chemotherapy and other medical treatments in mediating these features, all put it squarely within the area of concern of social policy and social work.

In any cross-cultural study there is a need to find an analytical framework which does justice to individuality without forcing an alien construction or value judgement on a particular system; or treating each system as individualistic to the point of eccentricity or exoticism. Anthropologists make a distinction between etic analysis (using an imposed frame of reference) and emic analysis (working within the conceptual framework of those studied) (Harris, 1979, 1987).

Both modes of understanding are vital if the unique qualities of the Chinese system are to be appreciated and yet placed in a wider context that permits a more scientific analysis. Thus concepts from the West have been used to explicate the Chinese experience. It is unfortunate that no emic accounts of any depth have been written by Chinese psychiatrists. Although the persecution to which intellectuals were subjected during the Cultural Revolution have come to an end, scholars and practitioners are still very wary of committing to paper any views which might be considered by those in power to be controversial.

To what extent do ideology, history and the economy influence the delivery of services to mentally ill people? Is there a wider 'truth' about societal reactions to mental illness that does not depend on ideology and may be found across cultures? Any reader familiar with the history of the development of mental health services and the treatment of mentally ill people in Western countries will find much in what follows wholly familiar. I have assumed that readers will not need to have these comparisons drawn constantly to their attention as such an approach would become tedious. Yet, naturally, it is diversity that catches the attention. For instance, one of the unique features in the Chinese system is the overt involvement of ideology and politics in the thinking of ordinary people. An example of this comes from an essay written for me by one of the patients at the hospital I studied.

> "Parents must be very sad when they face their crazy sons and daughters and find that they are helpless. Fortunately, the great, glorious and correct Chinese Communist Party, the great People's Republic of China, they loved and cared for the crazy sons and daughters down to the very last detail. They sent the crazy sons and daughters to the mental hospital for treatment" (Essay 29).

The study reported here starts with an historical perspective, outlining the development of modern psychiatric services in China since the opening of the first psychiatric hospital in 1898, through the post-Liberation period after 1949, and the Cultural Revolution, to the beginning of the 1980s. Many of the ideas about the treatment of those suffering from a mental illness were brought into China from outside: either from America and Europe before 1949 or from Russia after that date. For the Chinese, there is an uncomfortable tension between wishing to have techniques that are effective, and at the same time resisting the dominance of Western psychiatric theories, as they try to develop "psychiatry with Chinese characteristics".

Chapter 2 is concerned with aspects of the law that pertain to those with a psychiatric illness, and the rights that such people have. One of the major themes running through the provision of psychiatric services in China is the need to protect the wider community from the socially disruptive behaviour of mentally ill people. The balance of concern favours the collective over the individual and therefore emphasises social control rather than self-actualisation, an attitude which is consistent with other facets of Chinese society. There are no legal protections from involuntary admission for psychiatric patients and the decision to admit rests with the family and the doctors. On its own terms, Chinese law treats mentally ill offenders 'leniently', with a hospital disposal accepted as a more humane outcome than imprisonment for those who are particularly socially disruptive.

Chapter 3 discusses policy continuities and developments in both the health and welfare fields as they affect the provision of services for people with a mental illness. A comparative framework is delineated in which Chinese and Western solutions to the common problems faced in the provision of welfare are examined.

The experience of mental illness outside the confines of the hospital for both patients and relatives is dealt with in Chapter 4. As is the case in other countries, it is the families of mentally ill people who bear the main responsibility for looking after them. The difference in China is that they have much less assistance in performing their tasks than might be the case in Western countries. There are few, if any, non-governmental organisations or pressure groups to provide a range of services and support (Pearson & Phillips, 1994*a*). Chinese examples of family intervention are discussed, as is the range of services that constitute the Chinese model of community care.

The Chinese are aware of the advantages of providing care for psychiatric patients outside institutions, not least because it is held to be cheaper than providing beds for the millions of people who suffer from mental illness. It probably would be fair to say, however, that the Chinese would cite a lack of hospital beds as the major problem they face. It is not that China lacks a coherent and integrated theoretical model of community care (Pearson, 1992*a*; Phillips *et al*, 1994). The problems lie in implementing this model throughout the vast area of China. Difficulties centre around a paucity of resources, the lack of trained staff, the decline of the culture of voluntarism (Chan & Chow, 1992; Chan, 1993) and an environment which is generally inhospitable to people with a mental illness. Unfortunately, as in most other countries, the gap between the rhetoric and reality of community care is enormous, with the heaviest burden falling on families.

The remainder of the book is concerned with an empirical study of one psychiatric hospital (the Municipal Hospital discussed in Chapter 5) that mainly cared for patients diagnosed as suffering from chronic schizophrenia. I have decided to name neither the hospital nor its locality. All personal names have been changed as well as a few other details that would provide clues to location.

The reader might like to have some idea of how typical the Municipal Hospital is of psychiatric hospitals in China as a whole and here the answer can only be tentative. It has to take into account not only the size of the country but in particular the differences between rich and poor provinces. In comparison with the range of standards over the country as a whole, this hospital is probably slightly above average, but is not in the same class as the premier hospitals in Shanghai and Beijing. However, in a sense, it is the more interesting because of that, being more typical of the ordinary psychiatric hospital in China.

The possibility for data collection at the Municipal Hospital came about as a result of a programme of academic and professional exchange between the hospital and a non-governmental organisation in Hong Kong providing community based services for people recovering from psychiatric illness. Such programmes are becoming increasingly common and are part of the integration of Hong Kong and China as 1997 approaches.

My Chinese language skills are extremely limited and it was clear from the start that I would have to work through an interpreter/assistant. This person would need to be knowledgeable about mental health matters, fluent in both Chinese and English and able to handle the very delicate matter of translating not only the words but the spirit of a communication. Two of my own ex-graduate students in social work, both practising social workers who met these criteria, agreed to accompany me. In addition,

relevant written material in Chinese was translated into English for my benefit.

I have attempted to examine the hospital from the perspectives of both the patients and the staff. Fielding & Fielding (1986) advise selecting at least one method that is specifically suited to exploring the structural aspects of the research area and at least one that captures the essential elements of meaning for those involved.

The study of the Municipal Hospital included quantitative material based on information from patients' files. The hospital leaders were requested to prepare a list of all patients diagnosed as suffering from schizophrenia between the ages of 16 and 60. From the 460 names that this produced, a one in three random sample was drawn, giving a total of 150 patients. The data collection forms were prepared in Hong Kong and amended by hand at the hospital, when it became apparent that some of the expected information was mostly not available (for instance on the patient's family background), while unexpected data (for instance on educational and occupational attainment) was included.

Attempting to explore the world of meaning for staff and patients proved rather more difficult. This aspect was approached through an essay competition for the patients and interviews of both patients and staff, combined with ward observation. It would be disingenuous to pretend that my previous experience of psychiatric hospitals did not colour my perception of the Municipal Hospital. At the same time, strenuous efforts were made to avoid imposing on the data categories of cultural meaning derived from the West.

Chapter 5 contains a description of the hospital, the setting, staffing, financing, management policies, and total patient population. The results of data collected from the patients' files are examined in Chapter 6, followed in Chapter 7 by the results of an opportunity for patients to speak with their own voices, through excerpts from both the interviews and the essays that some patients wrote in response to the essay competition. This was done in an effort to provide a means through which patients could choose whether or not to express personal experiences and feelings without any pressure, in a way that would not be influenced by predetermined categories set by the research worker.

This book is an attempt to understand the complexity of the experience of psychiatric illness in China and the facilities that exist to 'serve the people' who suffer its consequences – a challenging task. This has not been attempted before by a foreigner (or, as far as I know, by a Chinese person), and is thus the first, and not the last, word on this fascinating and enormous topic.

1 The development of psychiatric services in China

Chinese medicine has a history dating back many thousands of years. During that time theories were formulated about psychiatric disturbances and doctors treated patients accordingly, leaving meticulously observed case histories for future generations. *The Yellow Emperor's Classic of Internal Medicine (Huang-ti nei-ching su-wen)*, compiled during the second and first century BC describes a condition known as *kuang* which is generally accepted as acute psychotic excitement although a differentiation between mania, schizophrenia or organic psychosis is not made:

> "When the illness is grave the patient always takes off his garments and walks away, or ascends heights, chanting songs or even refuses to eat for several days. The patients can also climb over walls and roofs which were beyond his usual capacity".
> (Tien Jukang, 1985, p. 69)

Another psychiatric disorder, *dian*, was also recognised, the associated symptoms being lethargy and apathy. Tsang (1973*b*) points out that mental disorders in the East and West tended to be recognised in the same sequence, if not at the same time; epilepsy, then psychosis with excitement. Depression, *dian*, was not recognised until considerably later. Tseng suggests that this was because quiet people were well tolerated and accepted in China.

There appear to have been few books on mental disorders. Tien Jukang (1985) states that one was written by Zhang Jinyue in the seventeenth century called *Methods of Curing Mental Illness*. Liu Xiehe (1981) states that a special manual of prescriptions for treating psychosis was compiled before the first century AD but

8

was lost. Other than this, he denies the existence of any other books on the subject. Before the end of the nineteenth century and the introduction of Western medicine psychiatric symptoms were seen as an integral part of general medicine as practised by general doctors.

There was no tradition of institutional care for mentally ill people in imperial China. Needham (1970) reports that a few general hospitals were in existence before the Ming dynasty but the concept never really took root. Nor did the Chinese pharmacopoeia include medicines that were particularly effective in the symptomatic treatment of psychotic disorders, although there were, and are, preparations that have a sedative effect. Psychiatry, based as it is on an assumption that there are diseases of the mind, did not find fertile soil in the holistic medical traditions of China. Thus the introduction of asylums for the insane and the various forms of treatment that were espoused from that time may be seen as alien forms grafted onto Chinese society rather than an indigenous product.

Before the People's Republic

Since considerable detail concerning this period is available elsewhere (Pearson, 1991), an outline of the most salient points will be provided here. The first recorded psychiatric hospital in China was opened in Guangzhou in 1898. It is possible that there may have been an earlier one in Foshan in the same province, Guangdong, but no records remain.

The hospital was located in an area of Guangdong called Fangcun (more usually written as Fong Tsuen in older records) but was commonly known as Kerr's Refuge for the Insane, after its founder, John Kerr. Dr Kerr was an American medical missionary who had spent most of his adult working life in Guangzhou as the physician-in-charge of the Canton Hospital, the first hospital to be opened by missionaries in China (Tucker, 1983; Spence, 1980).

For many years Dr Kerr had been trying to persuade the Board of Missions of the American Presbyterian Church, who funded the Canton Hospital, to permit him to open a hospital for the mentally disturbed. They had always resisted his efforts, saying that he was already too heavily burdened. Possibly another cause of their reluctance was that they did not want the missionary medical effort to be 'tainted' by proximity to such a highly stigmatised and despised group of patients. Unlike surgery, and to some extent medicine, Western psychiatry at that time had little to offer China

in the way of clear therapeutic advances. There seemed to be a general agreement that caring for the insane would do little to enhance either the evangelistic opportunities or the reputation of the missionary societies within China.

Dr Kerr was not a man to be thwarted. On his retirement from the Canton hospital in his seventies, he spent most of his life savings and bought four acres of land on which Kerr's Refuge was built, with the aid of an anonymous Chinese donor who supported his vision. Kerr lived long enough to see the hospital opened and on his death his work was taken up by another medical missionary, Charles Selden, who had recently arrived in China. Kerr's third wife, Martha Noyes Kerr, continued to work at the hospital. It is a mark of the esteem in which the hospital was held during this period that on the occasion of her 84th birthday in 1924, Dr Sun Yat Sen (father of the first Chinese Republic, who at this time had intimate connections with Canton) sent her a message expressing his:

> "...gratification to learn that you attain today the great age of 84 years and sends you his best wishes and in the name of our people, thanks you for the good work that you have done in our midst". (Personal communication from Mrs Kerr's great nephew, Henry Noyes, quoting from family documents).

Under Selden's regime treatment at the Refuge consisted of an humanitarian approach (occupation, recreation, freedom within the hospital grounds, respect for patients) combined with drugs, cold baths and ingenious devices of his own invention for physical restraint (Selden, 1905; 1909). This was, more or less, accepted treatment by the international standards of the time.

The hospital seemed to meet a need locally. For the first six years it operated as a private institution and then agreed to take 'police cases', whose fees were paid from the public purse. By 1933 the hospital had expanded to 700 beds (Lamson, 1934). The missionary literature abounds with reports of ill-treatment of mentally ill people in the community (Ingram, 1918; McCartney, 1926; Woods, 1929; Kerr, 1898, Selden, 1905). Patients were described as being chained, or walled up in small rooms at home, beaten, their limbs deliberately broken to prevent them from being violent, burned as a form of exorcism and even, occasionally, killed by their families. Of course, the missionaries were not disinterested witnesses and the cases that came to their attention were likely to be those that were particularly difficult. Selden does comment, although less frequently, on the kindness family members might show to a relative with a mental illness. Yet, overall, the

situation of mentally ill people seems to have been wretched, a view confirmed by a Chinese psychiatrist with experience of working in China at that time (Wong, 1950). The first full-scale academic programme in psychiatry was established at the Peking Union Medical College (PUMC) in 1932 by Dr R. Lyman. Lyman stayed at PUMC until 1937, where he had a profound effect on the graduate training of psychiatrists. Many of China's current senior psychiatrists were students of his, or taught by his ex-students (Kleinman, 1986). Lyman encouraged the teaching of social work and sociology in his department at PUMC (Lyman, 1937; 1939). It was the department at PUMC that was at the forefront of academic research on neurology and psychiatry in China before 1949. Even so, psychiatry was still an unpopular subject. Kleinman (1986) points out that, despite Lyman's success in postgraduate training of psychiatrists at PUMC, only one graduate went into psychiatry out of the 116 graduates produced between 1924 and 1933.

The Chinese Society for Neurology and Psychiatry was formed in 1931 by two members of the PUMC (Kao, 1979). In Shanghai, the work in 1934 of Dr Fanny Halpern, trained in psychiatry in Vienna under Alfred Adler, led to new initiatives in teaching, research and practice.

Little is known about the extent of psychiatric provision before 1949 in China. Lamson (1934) reports that other than Kerr's Refuge there were no other separate psychiatric institutions in China, although there were psychiatric wards attached to general hospitals in Suzhou, Beijing and Shanghai. He claims that the Ministry of Justice announced its intention in 1930 to erect 'lunatic asylums' in various large cities but there is no evidence that this policy was ever carried out. By the time that the Communist Party came to power in 1949, Lin (1985a) states that there were five psychiatric hospitals and a small core of psychiatrists in Beijing, Shanghai, Nanjing, Guangzhou, Chengdu, Changsha and Harbin. All of these are places that had large foreign populations or significant foreign influence. Xia & Zhang (1981) offer a lengthier list: Guangzhou, Beijing, Shanghai, Nanjing, Shenyang, Suzhou, Dalian, Siping and Chengdu.

In an address to the American Psychiatric Association in 1948, Dr Karl Bowman reported on a three-month visit to China which he had undertaken on behalf of the World Health Organization to plan for the development of psychiatry and mental health there. He observed that China had very little psychiatry. By his estimates China at the time had approximately 600 psychiatric beds and less than 50 psychiatrists for a population of approximately 450 000 000 people. Treatment methods at the time of his report included insulin shock therapy, which he said was in use in virtually all psychiatric hospitals visited, as well as metrazol and what he referred to as 'electroshock treatment' (which presumably is electroconvulsive therapy and seems to be the first time that it is mentioned in any of the available literature).

Bowman described China's psychiatric facilities in the following terms:

> "The present psychiatric hospitals in China are poorly equipped and in a bad state of repair and are giving largely simple custodial care. Lack of money seems to be the most important reason for this condition and the psychiatric hospitals merely reflect the generally impoverished condition of China. The teaching of psychiatry in medical schools is badly handicapped by the fact that there are almost no teachers available. There is great interest in psychiatry and a desire to develop it in every way possible." (quoted in Kao, 1979, p. 47)

Tsung-yi Lin (a professor of psychiatry at the University of British Columbia and the Chinese government's first honorary adviser on mental health in the reform decade of the 1980s) makes the point that Western style psychiatry did not take root in China in the same way that was true for surgery and medicine. He attributes this to the greater language skill needed in teaching and demonstrating the subject to would-be learners; the fact that at that time there had not been similar breakthroughs in the treatment of mental illness comparable with the advances in the other branches of medicine; that psychiatry was more culture bound in its understanding of the human psyche and therefore less transferable. With regard to training:

> "Few medical students chose to specialize in psychiatry and even some of those who chose to do so had to overcome the strong objections of their parents to enter the speciality, which arose from their families' fear that the stigma attached to mental illness would be transferred to their members who intend to enter psychiatry and become psychiatrists". (Lin, 1985*a*, p. 5)

Croizier concludes that the philanthropy and humanitarianism of the best foreign medical institutions in China could not be separated from the worst features of Western imperialism. Even when they were stripped of their formal religious character and administration placed largely in Chinese hands, general policy and financial support remained in foreign hands. Ultimately, he says, "'the whole missionary humanitarian effort in China fell before the rising tide of revolutionary nationalism". (Croizier, 1975, p. 24).

The People's Republic: 1949–1966

The Communist government of the new People's Republic of China decided to sever all ties with the non-Communist countries of the Western world. The Soviet Union became the focus of scientific and cultural relations. Chinese psychiatry was cut off from the West at a time when radical improvements in psychopharmacology, diagnosis and neurobiological research were being made. This was particularly difficult for the small core of psychiatrists, all of whom were trained in Western theories and techniques.

Soviet psychiatry exerted a monopolistic influence on Chinese psychiatry. Following an influential conference held in China in 1953, Pavlovian theory was introduced as the dominant theory for understanding human behaviour. A well organised nation-wide movement was launched by the Ministry of Public Health and the Chinese Medical Association to encourage, or even coerce, all psychiatric professionals to learn Pavlovian theory, which dominated psychiatry until the end of the Cultural Revolution in 1978 (Lin, 1985a).

Psychology began to be viewed with suspicion as a means of accentuating individual differences. Intelligence testing and clinical psychology particularly were not encouraged (Chin & Chin, 1969). As Breger comments, looking back on this period:

> "Psychological testing points out individual differences and, according to the values of the Cultural Revolution, did not serve to integrate man into society". (Breger, 1984, p. 128)

Sociology and anthropology were also banned. This, among other things, has permitted a predominantly medical model of psychiatric practice to develop with little input from professionals with a background in the social sciences such as psychologists, social workers and occupational therapists.

Perhaps reflecting the importance that the new government gave to improving the health of the people, and possibly within the spirit of the times when almost anything seemed achievable in the new world, there appears to have been a great deal of enthusiasm among those engaged in psychiatric work. The Chinese Society of Neurology and Psychiatry was formed in 1954 and in

1955 began to publish *The Chinese Journal of Neurology and Psychiatry.*
There may also have been an element of nationalistic pride in the
determination to cast off Western 'superstitions' as Mao called
them, and to show what China could do unaided, exemplified by
this statement from the deputy director of the Ministry of Health
in 1958:

> "Our goal was to reach a satisfactory level in patient management
> within one to two years and the world's advanced standards in
> the scientific and technological aspects of psychiatry within two
> to three years. In time, the number of psychiatric patients in
> China would decrease". (Lin, 1985a, p. 11)

Wu (1959) writes that, especially after the Great Leap Forward
in 1958, medical workers

> "...realized that it is their responsibility to serve the patients
> well. Therefore, there was a suggestion in many mental hospitals
> to let the mental patients enjoy the real humane treatment of
> socialism and they should live the life of normal people".
> (quoted in Kao, 1979, p. 113)

We have observed Kerr's Refuge through Western eyes both at
its inception and through its early years. The last published
reference from its doctors was Selden (1937) who said that it had
had to close due to trouble from the "communistic labour unions".
We are able to meet it again, in the early 1950s, but this time from
the point of view of the Chinese. The situation prior to Liberation
in 1949 was described thus:

> "The hospital had only very few workers, proper doctors and
> nurses were even less. The facilities were very poor, people were
> inadequately fed and had not enough warm clothes to wear, the
> food was poor and inadequate. Serious illness resulted due to
> cold weather and malnutrition. Hygienic conditions were very
> bad... the death rate once reached 36.5 per cent. We cannot
> really say there was any treatment for the patients, other than
> iron cages and iron ropes. The number of patients had once
> reached 1000, even though only 300–400 could be
> accommodated. Many patients did not even have a bed. For
> many years there were only 3 or 4 doctors in the hospital. At one
> time, there was no doctor, only a general practitioner who came
> in when called." (Mo, 1959, p. 310)

While conditions were doubtless exacerbated by the Japanese
occupation, the civil war, and so on, it would hardly be surprising

if the Chinese felt no debt of gratitude to the foreigners who introduced the hospitals, or any desire to emulate their model.

Psychiatric resources

To indicate the increase in facilities that took place between 1949 and 1958 two sources are worth quoting at length. A document was published in 1959 called *A Collection of Theses on Achievements in Medical Science in Commemoration of the Tenth National Foundation Day of China.* It contained an essay by Wu Cheng-i on psychiatry. He says that:

> "Sixty-two new hospitals were built throughout the 21 provinces and autonomous regions, with a total number of beds fourteen times greater than before Liberation. In 1950 the number of beds in the psychiatric wards was 1.1 % of the total capacity and in 1957 it was 3.6 %. There are now quite a few psychiatric sanatoriums in various areas for the chronically ill. The hospital staff increased as more hospitals and more beds became available. The number of doctors in 1958 was sixteen times that in 1949. The increase in the number of nurses was twenty-fold". (reproduced in Kao, 1979, p. 110)

If only he had mentioned his baseline figures!

The next document is more specific, although the numbers do not entirely concur with those of Dr Wu. It was the Five Year Plan published in 1958 and known as *The Circular of the Ministry of Health Concerning the Issuance of the National Mental Illness Prevention Work Plan (1958–1962).* It states that there were about 1000 psychiatric beds at the time of the Liberation and 50 or 60 "mental disease specialists", although the document does not say what training they had received, if any. It continues:

> "According to incomplete statistics, there are now in China 46 mental hospitals and clinics with 11 000 beds in twenty-one provinces and municipalities and the number of professional personnel for mental illnesses has been increased to 5000 or more among which some 400 are doctors (including some 30 doctors of Chinese medicine). Ending in 1957, some 73 000 mentally ill persons were treated and among them some 27 000 recovered". (reproduced in Kao, 1979, p. 122)

Ho (1974, p. 624) quotes figures of 73 150 admitted and over 63 280 discharged but makes no mention of recovery.

There were very few resources available to establish and fund new facilities. The *Chinese Journal of Neurology and Psychiatry* from this period carries an article describing how one hospital was set up (Zutangshan Care and Education Home Staff, 1958). It may well have been included as a model to encourage the others. It concerns the establishment of a hospital for chronic mental patients who were originally vagrants in Nanjing. The authorities took over an old temple, 40 miles outside the city. There was no electricity, no running water and no transport access. As the authors say, "the hospital was established with the spirit to conquer difficulties". (p. 259)

It seems from the article that none of the eight cadres were doctors, although two of them were described as 'medical workers'; nor had they worked with psychiatric patients before. The rest of the staff, described as 'care-takers', were ex-residents of the Civil Affairs Bureau's facilities for the poor and sick. Not surprisingly, most of the 'care-takers' were frightened and reluctant, apparently armed for their task only with exhortations to develop "the spirit of running a hospital with hard work, economisation and the spirit to serve the patients with all your heart". (p. 260)

The article, while extolling the virtues of socialism in helping to overcome difficulties, is also very forthright about the fleas, the incontinence, and the painful learning that brought them to realise that their patients were happier when meaningfully occupied, when their opinions were sought, and when they had cultural and recreational activities in which to be involved. Much of the increase in facilities that China saw between 1949 and 1959 was probably along similar lines.

The Nanjing Conference

Another landmark event in the development of Chinese psychiatry was the First National Conference of Psychiatric Specialists at Nanjing in 1958. It was organised by the Ministry of Health and was attended by over 90 persons holding key positions in the field of mental health (Ho, 1974). The conference was influential in setting directions for mental health policy.

Most particularly, it advocated a move away from Western domination of theory and practice and towards developing indigenous texts, expressed in the slogan "destroy superstition, believe in ourselves". It focused on the need for collective action to overcome the problems of mentally ill people, manifested in a willingness to move out of the urban centres and to provide services in the rural areas, and condemned 'individualistic' practices; it demanded that practitioners move away from the use of restraint and explore ways of implementing dialectical materialist thought in the treatment of patients. Above all there was to be "no shrieking in the adult wards and no crying in the children's wards" (Ho, 1974; Chin & Chin, 1969).

Not everyone agreed with the adoption of these new principles and apparently there were heated debates at the conference about the advisability of giving up the use of restraints and mechanical treatments. One has to bear in mind that at the time there was very little else, so it was tantamount to asking doctors to give up virtually all practices that were familiar to them, and to substitute a form of political education in which none of them had experience and for which there was no existing proof of efficacy. These doctors argued that locking up patients was for their own good. This rationale was criticised as being 'capitalistic' in its orientation. Shen Yucun wrote:

> "After great debates... the restraining of patients was finally abolished; wards were completely opened, thus breaking the traditional system of locking up psychiatric wards of the past hundreds and thousands of years. Patients have been liberated." (1958, p. 347)

At the conference, difficulties impeding progress were discussed. It was apparently still difficult to recruit suitable staff. There was an unwillingness to take up mental health work because it was seen as a low status job that carried a high risk of being attacked or verbally abused by patients.

The Five Year Plan, 1958–62

The national Five Year Plan of 1958 turned out to be the only five year plan dealing with mental health matters for many years. As such it is worth closer examination. It began by stating:

> "Mental illness is one in which the higher nervous activities of the human body are chaotic and there is a mental block. It brings not only pains and distress to the patient but also brings certain perils to industrial and agricultural production as well as social security".

Thus, a quasi-Pavlovian explanation of mental illness which did little to enlighten was put forward. The unpleasant nature of the illness for the sufferer was acknowledged but more concern was expressed about the economic consequences for the nation and the effect people with a mental illness could have on public order and safety. The authors of the plan acknowledged that many people with a mental illness did not receive any or proper treatment and were not necessarily well cared for at home. They estimated that 200 per 100 000 of the population in China were suffering from a mental illness.

The authors of the plan were critical about the macro-level of health organisation which concentrated too many resources on "what is new, what is big and what is regular", which is to say Western, at the expense of looking at cheaper, more efficient and effective solutions to service provision. The plan also pointed out that such authorities focused too much on hospital based services and too little on providing out-patient facilities and early and preventive treatment.

Hospital managers were criticised for caring more about the convenience of the staff than the comfort of the patients. Some of them were said to have lacked professionalism, and it was claimed that there were "still some working personnel who dislike patients, discriminate against them and despise them". The report suggested that managers should not automatically assume that patients cannot have an opinion worth listening to, and should take their wishes and suggestions into account. It is impossible not to be struck by the relevance that these strictures have for many psychiatric hospitals in the West!

The report advocated the following:

(a) Three kinds of organisational pattern; a medical base, a preventive unit and sanatoria (for chronic care)

(b) Caring for people in their homes or sending them to rural areas where there was a need for labour (this idea seems to have been predicated on the notion that rural living would be less stressful, although it is hard to imagine that the patient used to an urban environment might find it so)

(c) Four kinds of cure; by Chinese and Western medicines and physical therapy; by proper labour therapy; therapy through organised sports and cultural amusements; and systematic educational therapy. These four principles continue to be the major therapeutic guidelines.

With regard to treatment, the plan emphasised the need to "summarise and propagate seriously the clinical experiences of Chinese medicine". It categorically forbade frontal lobotomy or other clinical methods that could "injure the lives and health of the patients... binding or imprisoning of patients must be resolutely opposed".

The establishment of 'mental disease sanatoria' and 'mental disease convalescent villages' were also mooted, which at least by implication seemed to be intended for chronic patients. These were expected to be at least partially self-supporting through agricultural, light industrial and handicraft work. Sanatoria and villages are also mentioned by Chao (1965) but they do not appear to be a significant part of services in the 1980s or '90s (Jin & Li, 1994). Each province was supposed to establish a regional hospital centre, for the guiding of preventative work and the training of personnel. Joint planning involving 'three men leading groups' was to be set up with representatives of local health, civil affairs and public security bureaux to coordinate activities. This continues to be the mechanism by which mental health services are currently planned, implemented and coordinated in the People's Republic of China (PRC).

Building of more hospitals as the solution to problems of mental ill health was not envisaged in the plan. Consistency with the government's approach to physical ill-health may be observed in the encouragement to provide more out-patients' facilities and to provide some beds in local general hospitals.

Six regional collaborative centres were established in Beijing, Nanjing, Chengdu, Changsha, Guangzhou and Shanghai. These regional centres were to be responsible for training personnel, particularly at the middle levels to work in treatment and prevention of mental illness. They were also to train administrative cadres and to undertake research and in general to become centres of excellence. In their studies they were to "adopt the communist working style of imagination, outspokenness and daring". While we may find ourselves out of sympathy with the political rhetoric that accompanies these ideas, the ideas themselves represent high standards of practice. It would, of course, be unwise to assume that these standards were necessarily translated into action, but this is only one more feature of common experience that China shares with the rest of the world.

The Cultural Revolution

The Cultural Revolution is generally dated as having lasted from 1966 to 1976, with the worst excesses in the first four years. Politics took command with a vengeance. Schools and universities were closed. Intellectuals and professionals were vilified and frequently sent down to work on communes, leading to the closure of some hospitals and/or a great diminution in the services they could offer.

Naturally, this had an effect on the psychiatric services although it is by no means easy to determine precisely what this was. Before discussing the detail of what is known, the intellectual and political environment in which these reports were produced must be examined. Other than the documents previously mentioned, almost everything that is known about the Cultural Revolution period as it affected psychiatry is based on verbal reports given to visiting Westerners. There are no statistics, policy statements or research to guide us.

Consequently, it is imperative to distinguish between facts and normative statements made by Chinese colleagues (Lin, 1985a). Kleinman & Mechanic (1979) point out that although it was widely reported that the use of binding and isolation had been banned in psychiatric hospitals, they observed locked isolation rooms and patients bound hand and foot during a visit to a teaching institution. Careful reading of the literature also finds references to the continuing use of ECT, despite its supposed ban after 1959: in Changsha (Brayfield, 1978); in Guangzhou (Kraft & Swift, 1978); in Nanjing (Walls *et al*, 1975).

Lin (1985a) goes on to say that a model project is often mistaken by a visitor for a typical one. He suggests this may be due either to language difficulties or over-zealousness by the speaker in emphasising points to the visitor. A third factor may also be involved; the visitor's willingness to believe what he/she is told because it is what he wants to hear, as:

> "In Hangzhou a cadre explained how easy it had been in 1972 to convince me – as he himself had done – that all was well, even wonderful, in school, factory and commune. We 'foreign friends', plainly were sitting ducks. 'I wanted to deceive you' he said 'but you *wanted* to be deceived." (Jonathan Mirsky, quoted in Brown, 1981, p. 9)

This issue is important in looking at the reports by Western visitors that were published between 1964 and 1980. For a number of years, from 1949 to about 1971, reports by foreigners on China's psychiatric services based on an actual visit were extremely rare (Lazure, 1964; Thompson *et al*, 1967; Chin & Chin, 1969). Cerny (1965) is much quoted, but he synthesized material from existing sources, including Russian material, and does not appear to have visited China himself.

It was only after the beginning of 'ping pong' diplomacy and the start of a rapprochement with the United States that foreign visitors again were permitted to visit. These visitors tended to be those like the Sidels (Sidel, 1973; Sidel & Sidel, 1973, 1982) who were known to have a sympathy towards communism, members of delegations who were known 'friends of China', like the Society for Anglo-Chinese Understanding (Adams, 1972), or academic visitors with a particular professional interest (Sainsbury, 1974). Reading through over 30 reports dating from this time it is quite clear that they are based on very restricted information and are biased either by lack of knowledge (which is hardly surprising considering the closed nature of the country in the previous 15 to 20 years), or because of the writer's own political sympathies.

Again this is not surprising. China is ultra-sensitive to criticism and would have been more likely to grant permission to visitors who were likely to offer support. Even now, it is not possible to write about China without being aware of how what is published will be received by the Chinese authorities, and how this will in turn affect future access, not only for oneself but for others.

It is all too easy to be knowing after the event. Even so, reading some of these reports, it does seem that these Western visitors left their critical and analytical faculties at home to an extent not called for by the circumstances. Leung *et al* (1978, p. 355) comment that:

> "If one took away concerns about money and debt, about success in the eyes of peers and parents, about love and jealousy, about the success of one's children and about 'what is the meaning of my life', caseloads in North America might drop considerably."

They seem willing to ignore the potential effects of many aspects of Chinese society at that time on the wellbeing of its citizens. Examples would include mandatory late marriages; in-law tensions; involuntary geographical separation of married people; allocated jobs rather than ones reflecting interest, ability or preference; fierce public criticism sessions leading to intense humiliation; being sent down to work in a commune and losing your right to live in your home town; to say nothing of the environment of chaos, suspicion and insecurity created by the Cultural Revolution.

A close examination of the literature soon reveals that the vast majority (although not all) of the foreign observers were reporting on the same two hospitals: the Shanghai Number One and the Beijing Medical College Third Hospital. The reports enjoy a certain consistency because they are based on the same statements by the same doctors.

Not only were these probably the top two hospitals in the country, but because of their location they were very close to the political heartland. Thus Brown (1980) points out that Shanghai was very much influenced by the Gang of Four, and this may explain why the policies reported at the Shanghai Number One

Hospital may have so closely followed the official line about not using ECT, binding and isolation. The two most influential doctors at the Beijing Medical College were Professor Wu Cheng-i and the psychiatrist-in-charge, Shen Yucun. Both doctors were referred to in the previous section. It was Professor Wu who was selected to write the essay on psychiatry to contribute to the collection on China's medical achievements since Liberation, to celebrate the tenth anniversary of the founding of the People's Republic. Shen Yucun's impassioned celebration of the banning of inhuman treatments as the policy at the Nanjing Conference of 1959 would suggest that any hospital of which she was in charge would not feature these methods of restraint. Neither of them could be considered typical either in ability or influence of the doctors working in hospitals in more remote provinces and centres. Thus Ho's assertion (1974, p. 133) that "the Chinese have been able to put these ideas into practice on a massive national scale within a relatively short period of time" seems at best unproven (and possibly unprovable).

The socialist model of psychiatry

With these sizeable caveats, what picture emerges of the state of psychiatry during the Cultural Revolution? Sidel describes in some detail the principles of revolutionary optimism that govern psychiatry. These are:
  (a) The feelings of the individual should be subordinated to the needs of the group of which he is a member – the family, the classroom, the commune, the entire society
  (b) The individual is part of something larger than himself, the revolution, and that this revolution will ultimately be victorious
  (c) The participation in an ultimately victorious revolution gives meaning and joy to life, even if the road to revolution is paved with personal sacrifice
  (d) People have an infinite capacity to learn, to modify their thinking, to understand the world around them and to remould themselves through faith in the revolution and for the sake of the revolution (Sidel, 1973).
Despite this, Sidel comments that:

> "The psychiatric hospitals were the only segment of Chinese life that we saw in which depression rather than exhilaration was the predominant affect." (1973, p. 732)

Karenga (1978) develops a five point model of Chinese psychosocial therapy. The first salient feature is the definition of the social dimensions of the problem. Thus the phenomena of mental illness are viewed largely as the product of the failure of the old political system. Solutions must be directed towards a sick society rather than a sick individual.

The second feature concerns the definition of the personal dimensions of the problem. Mental illness is seen as essentially problems in thought, and therapy as thought liberation. The individual expresses this as a rejection of reality and a refusal to accept the design and demands from a social context in which the patient feels alienated. At the same time, all individuals have the ability to learn and change both themselves and the world around them. Thus if the patient is informed of the correct way to view circumstances he/she can be encouraged to arm himself to fight his own illness. Ratner (1978, p. 82), who visited the Shanghai Number One Hospital, quotes one of the staff as saying:

"Chinese psychotherapy does not focus on the patient's emotions or childhood experiences; it does not attempt psychological explanations. The main concern is for the patients to develop logical, rational thinking and to develop good social values of cooperation. Then the patients can come to have happy, fulfilled lives through their ordinary social activities. In other words because social life is fulfilling, the point is to participate in it and there is no need to engage in purely psychological, personal analysis."

The major technique to help patients develop rational thought was the study of Mao's works, particularly *Where Do Correct Thoughts Come From?*, *On Contradictions* and the ones referred to as 'the three constantly read articles'. These were: *In Memory of Norman Bethune*; *To Serve The People*; and *The Foolish Old Man Who Could Move Mountains*. Staff were supposed to take the lessons contained in what are essentially allegorical tales and help patients to apply those lessons to their own lives.

In Western terms, this could be said to fit a model of cognitive therapy, couched in rational-directive terms. The political content is clearly a culturally specific feature. Because it seems such a strange way to approach the treatment of psychotic disorder to a Western observer, it has received much attention in the literature. Yet as a means of orienting the patient to a reality outside him or herself, of reminding him of a world other than his inner one and of reaching patients, many of whom would have been illiterate, it may have had some effectiveness. Leung *et al* (1978) give an example from a session at which they were present when an ex-patient came back to talk about her experiences. She related her personal oppression and mistreatment by her in-laws which led to her breakdown. Through group discussions of Chairman Mao's writings, she came to realise while in hospital that in the New China there was a guarantee of equality of the sexes and protection of individual rights. She claimed such knowledge motivated her to re-assert her own individual dignity and led to her liberation from in-law domination.

It is commonly accepted that the success of any particular therapeutic theory or method does not always lie in the nature of the method itself but in the therapist's enthusiasm and faith in the treatment which conveys itself to the patient. It is most unlikely that Mao's thoughts did much to control acute psychosis, but they may have had a part to play in what we would think of as the social rehabilitation of the patient.

This approach to the patient, as a conscious being with a capacity to learn and change, continues an ages old approach to human beings and their essential educability which is Confucian in origin. People were fundamentally good but behaved wrongly because of faulty understanding (Bodde, 1957). Thus they could be educated into better ways both by being presented with new ideas and with exemplars who would demonstrate the correct way to behave. This use of models is seen again and again in mass campaigns (Burch, 1979). The archetypal model is Lei Feng, who died after an accident as a young man, but not before he had declared that he wished no more than "to be a rustless screw in the machine of the revolution", and has been held up ever since as an exemplar of the model young citizen.

Hospitals in China since 1949 have tended to use the army as a model. Given that the concept of a hospital at all is a foreign one, a mode of conceptualising its organisation and functions based on something that is familiar is almost certain to be sought. The political climate and the imagery involved in revolution made the use of a military model almost inevitable. Wards were divided into 'fighting groups' with the positions of corporal and sergeant being taken by the model patients, known as the Red Sentries – patients on the road to recovery who were expected to set an example and to take care of newer and sicker patients (Ho, 1974; Frears, 1976; Lu, 1978).

The third aspect of Karenga's model is that of the collective solution at the levels of construction, concern and execution. Ho (1974) points out that individualism has very different connotations for the Chinese. Whereas in the West, it implies dignity, freedom, and responsibility, the Chinese view it as selfish or undisciplined action divorced from the group. Clearly, if mental illness is not seen as an individual problem then it is likely to be conceived as more amenable to a collective solution:

> "The hospital becomes not only a battle ground for struggling against illness but also a classroom for learning and practicing socialism." (Ho, 1974, p. 626)

The fourth feature is the collective implementation of therapeutic procedures, whereby the patient is not exempt from the responsibilities pertaining to an ordinary citizen, is expected to contribute to national reconstruction through labour, and to take part in political study groups. The passive patient is supposedly transformed into the aware and active participant of his or her own liberation and ultimately the liberation of society.

Finally comes the construction and maintenance of supportive relationships. The focus is shifted from the individual to the environment in which he or she lives and works. A network of supportive relationships are established and coordinated to keep the patient out of institutions where possible and in the community where treatment and support can take place in familiar settings. Thus Rosner (1976) reports from the Peking Medical College Third Hospital that staff teams made home and factory visits to prepare the way for the patient and to make sure that he or she was being offered suitable work on discharge.

Explaining mental illness

The aetiology of mental disorder contained some logistical problems for the Chinese during this time. As has already been discussed, there clearly was a tendency to think of causation in terms of social and class factors, although I can find no reference to any public declaration that mental illness could be eradicated through the implementation of a socialist society. There was perhaps a tendency to think that there would be a diminution as shown in the remarks by the deputy minister of health already quoted. This is a point also discussed by Kao (1974).

However, with the evidence before their eyes that the new China still had its quota of mentally ill people, social explanations of causation were hardly likely to be popular. It is one thing to argue that the injustices of capitalism drive people mad, but it requires a different order of thinking to examine the flaws in the Cultural Revolution that might contribute to mental disturbance. As a consequence of this, notions about aetiology are not well defined during this period.

Frears (1976, p. 21) quotes an article from the *China Pictorial* in 1971 which attempts to explain mental illness by saying that:

"A mental illness is different from an ideological illness. And to restore function of the cerebrum to normal, medicinal treatment is necessary. Although the cause of illness was different in each case most of the patients were in the grip of an intense mental struggle, or had lapsed into melancholia for a prolonged period owing to their inability to deal with the objective world correctly. Failure to free themselves of it caused the cerebrum to lose part of its function."

On the whole, this contributes little to our understanding.

Kety (1976) asked Professor Wu Cheng-i to describe his concept of schizophrenia. He said that he saw it as a disease of the brain, biochemically and physiologically, but with important components determined by life experience. A colleague of Professor Wu, Dr Yen, offered a very eclectic explanation that would be familiar to Western doctors. He said that he felt that schizophrenia is some kind of biochemical or physiological disturbance in the brain that also requires some experiential stress for its expression, but that stress is not enough since everyone with the same stress does not develop schizophrenia. He also feels that genetic predisposing factors may exist.

In Nanjing, when asked whether they believed in the developmental theory of mental illness (based on Freudian concepts), the psychiatrists there replied that they did not:

"Under Chairman Mao's guidance, after Liberation everyone believes in dialectical materialism and everyone is happy. There is no conflict for our children." (Walls *et al*, 1975, p. 124)

In the same article, Shanghai psychiatrists were reported as having answered the same question in the following way:

"We have not yet arrived at a unified explanation as to the causes of mental disease. Some people hold that the role is played by chemical changes in the brain or genetic factors. We think that a reasonable social system will reduce the environmental causes of mental diseases. But will it also be effective in reducing the occurrence of schizophrenia? Well, there are still some disputes." (Walls *et al*, 1975, p. 124)

An educational notice for patients posted on the wall in the same hospital said that:

"Psychosis is an illness which shows the abnormality of psychiatric activities. It can be brought on by various causes which have one thing in common, a functional disorder of the brain." (Brown, 1980, p. 26.)

There seems to have been a discrepancy in this issue when so much attention was paid in practice to social involvement and political understanding, while as Brown (1980) pointed out, research focused (as it still does) much more strongly on biochemical issues.

The 1980s – seeking truth from facts

The numbers of reports on Chinese psychiatry written by Western observers decreased markedly during the 1980s. This may have been because China had ceased to be quite so exotic to the West, so that the same intensity of interest was not generated by information on her psychiatric services and not so much material was offered or published. It may also have been balanced by the increasing numbers of articles available in English language journals written by psychiatrists from the People's Republic. Exchange projects like the one between the University of Washington and the Hunan Medical College in Changsha gave Chinese psychiatrists greater access to Western ideas and the chance to synthesize these ideas with their own experience.

Some of the characteristics that made China different, like the use of Mao's works in treatment, have clearly faded away. Masserman (1980), Bloomingdale (1980) and Achtenberg (1983) all comment on how this practice had ceased. There seemed to be a greater willingness on the part of Chinese psychiatrists to speak frankly. On the subject of Mao's thought, Dr Young Derson is quoted as saying:

"We do not believe that you can get a disease from a wrong idea – nor will a 'correct idea' cure a patient. We try to teach the meaning of illness, based on scientific knowledge." (Achtenberg, 1983, p. 373)

Some of the observers detect a lack of enthusiasm for the use of Chinese medicine in the treatment of schizophrenia. Parry-Jones (1986) says that its use continues, but appears to be regarded largely as an adjunct to Western methods and its efficacy seems to be viewed with some caution.

Breger (1984) failed to elicit strong support for acupuncture, particularly from those doctors trained in Western medicine. Tousley (1985) found no psychiatrists who recommended Chinese herbal medicine for psychosis although some used it as a means to ameliorate side-effects. Unlike the spirit of the 1970s when Western observers acted as ciphers of the official line, these newer reports have elements of evaluation, or even oblique criticism of some of the practices of which they were made aware. Euphemistically, Parry-Jones (1986) describes as 'interesting' the practice in Sichuan of using a particular herb to induce vomiting and seizures in cases of schizophrenia. Thornicroft (1987) describes as 'novel' the use of intravenous hydrocortisone in the treatment of childhood schizophrenia. Wilson & Hutchison (1983, p. 394) commented on the use of high doses of chlorpromazine which:

> "...precluded any emotional outbursts or disruptive behaviour. Keeping patients well-behaved, busy and compliant was acknowledged as a legitimate therapeutic goal by the staff. Patients sat quietly at long tables most of the day putting hairpins and metal snaps on cards. These activities were viewed as productive contributions to society."

ECT is widely reported as being given in unmodified form (Tousley, 1985; Parry-Jones, 1986; Thornicroft, 1987). The focus on physical treatment emphasises the lack of input from the social sciences that in the West has informed the treatment and understanding of mentally ill people and their families. This is demonstrated by the institutional nature of hospitals. They are bare, undecorated, completely devoid of any personal possessions belonging to the patients (Visher & Visher, 1979; Wilson & Hutchison, 1983; Parry-Jones, 1988; Priemus-Noach, 1988). Not even a photograph is to be seen. This is utterly unlike Chinese homes where even the poorest people have family photographs displayed and a calendar hanging on the wall. Homes are cluttered and filled by the lives of their inhabitants. None of this is apparent in a psychiatric hospital.

Conclusions

Psychiatry in China began as Western psychiatry. Its professional development mirrored practices in the West, and its practitioners were either foreigners or Chinese people trained in Western medicine. It did not root in an alien climate with the same vigour shown by medicine and surgery. As the twentieth century progressed psychiatry was increasingly at the mercy of the vagaries of an unstable political, economic and social environment.

From 1949, when the Communist Party came to power, there were more efforts to improve psychiatric facilities and to mould them into a more immediately recognisable Chinese shape. Politics interfered with what had been a promising beginning to lead psychiatry down a path that most would now seem to agree was a dead end.

The banning of psychology and sociology after the Liberation has had a long-term negative effect on the way that psychiatric care is offered. There is a lack of understanding about the way that the social milieu affects behaviour, and scant attention is paid to the personal psychological aspects which shape and form each individual's experience of psychotic illness.

The argument that the social system of the People's Republic reduces the incidence of mental illness is one that a number of Western visitors have found attractive. They seem temporarily to forget the freedoms, opportunities and comforts that make their own lives tolerable, and instead transform them into a burden. Thus they are able to admire the deprivation in others' lives as a moral virtue. An appreciation of socialism can only be honestly achieved by an holistic understanding of all its facets, and not by a process of selective blindness or wilful misunderstanding.

While the reports on psychiatry in China published since 1964 are of interest, they reflect the drawbacks of one-off visits and, in many cases, little understanding of China. Even those visitors who were on study tours that lasted six or eight weeks rarely stayed for long in one place. Informants were unlikely to see them again. There was no continuing relationship with the responsibility that this brings or the trust that gradually develops, both of these being particularly important in the Chinese context. Without this on-going relationship and ability to carry out research these reports provide little satisfaction.

My overall impression is that psychiatry in China has lost some of its sense of purpose and direction. Having been deprived of its guiding force of socialism in the 1950s and the more concentrated form of Maoism during the 1960s and 1970s, it has lost its prime organising principle. In this, it mirrors the forces at work in Chinese society during the last 12 years.

2 Mental illness, law and rights

Little is available in English that examines the way that China has viewed the legal status of those regarded as suffering from a mental illness, or how such people are dealt with when they transgress. As King & Bond comment:

> "In Western societies people struggle for rights, while in China, people are concerned with relationship construction." (1985, p. 41)

Ideas about the rule of law, equality for all before the law, and even justice, have traditionally been very different in China from those in Western countries (Hansen, 1985). Confucian thinking concentrated on the idea of *li*, proper behaviour, encouraging the belief that if every one knew his or her role and carried out the behaviour associated with it, then harmony would reign. This was tempered by the idea of *ren*, benevolence or human-heartedness. If Western law tried to be guided by consistency and logic, then *li* and *ren* required that law was subsidiary to flexibly interpreted custom and moral tradition (Bodde, 1957).

Citizens did not so much enjoy rights as hope to be ruled justly by a beneficent Emperor and his officials. When they were disappointed, as they frequently were, they had little official recourse. For millennia, the Chinese have lived with the knowledge that it is who you know that is truly important; thus the emphasis on building relationships.

An examination of Chinese records relating to law and mental illness suggests a coherence with other facets of Chinese thought in the emphasis given to the importance of maintaining social order rather than the preservation of individual freedoms. The concern of mental health practitioners in the West with the human rights of psychiatric patients finds no echo in China. What is the historical relation between law and mental illness in China? What is the current situation? How do the Chinese look at the question of human rights? Do they use mental hospitals to incarcerate political dissidents?

Before communism

According to Liu Xiehe (1981), the first mention of psychosis in the law was by Han Feizi (280–233 BC) who wrote that "psychotics cannot escape from punishment according to the law". From the later Han period onwards, representatives of the law tried to control psychotic outbursts. The first law directed at *kuang* sufferers was promulgated in AD 100 (Han dynasty). Such people were held sufficiently responsible for their actions to merit a penalty being set; but out of compassion for those who acted when they were not really themselves, the sentence was reduced (Chiu, 1981). However, it was only from the first half of the Qing dynasty that a sustained effort was made to eliminate such disruptions of the social order by using legislation to shift the responsibilities of family, community and officials towards those with a mental illness (Bunger, 1950; Chiu, 1981).

A continuing theme of concern of authors writing on this subject is whether and/or why Chinese law showed clemency to mentally ill offenders. The legal tradition of clemency in China for certain categories of offender evolved during the Zhou period (1122–770 BC) when the concept of the 'three pardonables' was developed to ensure the lenient treatment of offenders who were very young, or very old, or who were 'mentally incompetent'. These ideas were embodied in the Tang Codes (AD 618–907) which provided for relatively light sentences for those who suffered incurable diseases or those who were seriously ill. People with a mental illness were included in the latter category (Ng, 1980, 1990). The Qing Code dealing with the special conditions pertaining to youth, age and infirmity is almost identical to the relevant section of the Tang Code (Bodde, 1980).

Why were these people treated more leniently than other offenders? Bodde suggests two reasons. First, on the pragmatic grounds that they were not considered to be habitual criminals and were thought less likely to offend again. Second, and perhaps more important, because of a tradition of humanitarianism going back to Confucius. The Tang Code explains why, for instance, monetary redemption may properly be granted to wrongdoers who are aged, young or infirm by frequently introducing the words 'compassion' and 'love' into its discussion. The Tang commentary on the Code supports its argument by quoting a passage from the Book of Rites:

> "A person of eighty or ninety is called a venerable greybeard. A person of seven is called a child deserving of pity. A child deserving of pity and a venerable greybeard, even though they may have committed a crime, are not to be subjected to punishment." (quoted in Bodde, 1980, p. 140)

The Tang Code gave legal recognition to mental ailments as valid criteria for determining infirmity and incapacity. Two degrees are specified; 'feeble-mindedness' under infirmity and 'insanity' under incapacity. In Tang times, the feeble-minded and the insane were not held legally responsible for their actions, a situation which apparently persisted at least through the Song dynasty (960–1279).

The Qing Code employs a single generalised term, mental illness, which is discussed in relation to homicide but no other crimes (Bodde, 1980). The Qing homicide laws, which dictated lighter penalties for those with a mental illness, at least in relation to single homicides, may be seen within this tradition of clemency. They represented the view that an insane person lacked the capacity to reason, and was not aware of what he or she was doing and could not therefore be said to be guilty in the same way as other offenders. However, the punishments regarding multiple homicides committed by insane persons were draconian. The tradition of clemency was overridden because the enormity of multiple homicide and the threat it constituted to social order demanded punitive action, whatever the mental state of the defendant.

Bunger (1950) and Bodde (1980) point out that the emphasis on clemency fights a losing battle with the concern for social order throughout the Qing period. This is demonstrated by the registration and confinement laws for insane people that were introduced in 1689 (Chiu, 1981). Insane men were to be given into the custody of their families only if the authorities were satisfied that they could be locked up at all times. Insane women were automatically returned to their families after they had been registered. To assist families in their task, the government issued locks and fetters. Alabaster (1899, p. 53), writing in the late Qing period, noted:

> "Relatives are bound to report cases of lunacy and exercise strict supervision over the lunatics, under penalty of eighty blows with heavy bamboo if the lunatic kills himself, and one hundred blows if he kills anyone else... Lunatics are required to be

manacled and the relations must not remove the manacles without proper authority."

In practice, the registration law was difficult to enforce, because families often refused to register a family member with a mental illness. Neighbours and relatives were reluctant to intervene and busy magistrates gave the issue no priority. The demand for registration contravened centuries of pervasive wariness of becoming entangled with the law and its officials as well as standards of family loyalty and affection (Ng, 1980). Although the intention of the registration and confinement laws was to ensure public security rather than punish, it is unlikely that those affected by them were able to make such fine distinctions. The relevant sub-statute was repealed in 1908 (Ng, 1980).

Developments in the communist era

Jural law or societal law?

Leng & Chiu (1985) distinguish between the jural (formal) and societal (informal) models of law in China. Jural law is represented by codified rules, enforced by a judicial hierarchy. Societal law focuses on socially approved norms and values, inculcated by political socialisation and enforced by extra-judicial apparatus consisting of administrative agencies and social organisations. Leng & Chiu attribute the domination of societal law to Mao's bias against bureaucratisation. Others (Copper *et al*, 1985; Nathan, 1986*a*) also suggest that Mao saw law as a potential brake on the Revolution and an encumbrance to what Baum (1986) recognises as his preference for 'the rule of man'. The concept of the rule of man in China goes back to Confucius, who advised that a ruler and his subjects should be guided by the rules of *li*, ethics or proper behaviour, rather than by codifications of law. Behaviour should be mediated by moral principle rather than by the fear of punishment. In a different context, Mao also espoused this dictum, in fact if not in rhetoric. The principle is expressed in a 1960s Guangzhou Red Guard Pamphlet:

> "The principle of law is to develop fully the power of the proletarian dictatorship so that we can attack the enemy more effectively and more accurately; it may never be used to restrict the functioning of dictatorship. If we respectfully follow Chairman Mao's instructions, we are then following the highest principles of law." (Baum, 1986, p. 83)

Consequently, it was not until 1979 that China had a formal Criminal Law. Before 1979, it was impossible for the populace to know with any precision whether or not a particular action would be in breach of the law. The notion from the Napoleonic Code, that there should be no crime without a law (*nullum crimen, nulla poena sine lege*) adopted by Russia, found few supporters in China. Instead, the ancient Chinese principle of 'judgment by analogy' was reasserted in Article 79 of the Criminal Law. This stipulated that:

> "A crime not specifically proscribed under the specific provisions of the present law may be confirmed a crime and sentence rendered in light of the most analogous article under the special provisions of the present law." (Baum, 1986, p. 87)

The Lawyers' Committee for Human Rights (1993) points out that the use of analogy violates international legal standards against *ex post facto* laws. However, they claim that most lawyers in China favour maintaining this principle.

The ascendancy of the societal model over the jural model of law led to the complete dominance of the Party and the police in the administration of justice. This habit was far too deeply ingrained to be very much affected by the Criminal Law or Criminal Procedure Law of 1979. A 1981 law college textbook states:

> "Legislation must take party policy as its basis and administration of the law must take party policy as its guide. When legal provisions are lacking, we should manage affairs in accordance with party policy. When legal provisions exist they should be accurately applied, also under the guidance of party policy... Policy occupies the leading position... Law serves to bring policy to fruition." (Nathan, 1986*b*, p. 133.)

In 1985 an article in the *Beijing Review* (11 February 1985, p. 4), by An Zhiguo bemoaned the fact that party leaders in many places continued to think that the Party exercised leadership over everything, substituting party leadership for administration and regarding their own words as law.

The police, in the form of the Public Security Bureau, take a much more active role in dealing with wrongdoers than is the case elsewhere. It is a tradition that Chinese people on the whole prefer to avoid the adversarial context of a law court, and are willing to accept mediation or other means of settling disputes or minor crimes.

The police have very wide ranging powers to deal with minor offenders, political dissidents and socially undesirable or disruptive elements not charged with felonies (Copper *et al*, 1985; Baum, 1986; Edwards, 1986). Such people may be sent to camps and assigned to hard labour for periods up to four years and as they are defined as being subject to 'education' they are not entitled to public trial or legal counsel because technically they are not being punished. Re-arrests and re-assignments are permitted – in effect this is indeterminate detention without trial and without necessarily having committed a crime. With the passing of the Administrative Litigation Law in 1990, it is now theoretically possible to appeal against re-education through labour. No successful outcome has been reported in the few cases where this is known to have been attempted (Lawyers Committee for Human Rights, 1993).

There is no presumption of innocence (Leng & Chiu, 1985; Nathan, 1986*a*). Once an individual is in a court, it is almost certain that a guilty verdict will be returned. Baum (1986) claims that conviction rates are well over 90%. Copper *et al* (1985), based on a review of sentences in cases reported in two national and two provincial newspapers between the years 1978–1983, report that the highest proportion to be acquitted was 2.2% in 1981.

Currently, there is no comprehensive mental health law that covers all of China. The necessity for such a law is acknowledged. Wu Jiasheng (1985, p. 43) says:

> "Legislation and regulation for protection of social order against mental illness should be formulated soon. It seems that at the moment, the most outstanding problem is compulsory custodial treatment. For example, there are no clear guidelines to define the boundary, operational procedures, treatment means, period of detention for compulsory custodial treatment. There are also no clear guidelines regarding rights of the mental patients. From the perspective of a healthy socialist legislation, it is necessary to formulate these regulations."

Mental health legislation had been drafted and was expected to go before the 1990 National People's Congress. However, it was withdrawn at the last moment, and it may be some years before such legislation is officially ratified. The 1990 *Law of the People's Republic of China on the Protection of Disabled Persons* includes mentally ill people, thus affording them some degree of positive recognition (Tian *et al*, 1994). At the moment, laws affecting those with a mental illness are scattered through a wide variety of statutes.

Mentally ill offenders and the law

Criminal responsibility

The Chinese Criminal Law reflects the historic concern with the issue of diminished responsibility and clemency (Cohen & Gelatt, 1984, p. 14). Article 15 of the Law states:

> "A mental patient who causes harmful results when in a situation of being unable to understand or control his actions does not bear criminal responsibility. However, his family members or guardians should be instructed to keep close watch over him and give him medical treatment. A patient of intermittent insanity who committed offences when he was sane should bear criminal responsibility. A drunken person who committed offences should bear criminal responsibility."

The issue of what constitutes criminal responsibility, and how it is to be judged, is a central one for Chinese authors addressing the relationship between insanity and law. The offender's ability to understand his or her illegal act before and after the crime is committed does not pertain to the ruling of criminal responsibility, although it may have some bearing on the verdict (Beijing Medical University, 1986). The decision as to whether the offender should bear criminal responsibility is based on whether or not he had the capacity to do so at the moment the crime was committed. Although it is never stated as such, the question of intent (*mens rea*) seems to lie at the root of the arguments about the issue of responsibility (Hart, 1968).

Article 14 of China's Criminal Law implies that persons under the age of 16 are assumed to have no criminal responsibility, except in the case of very severe crimes committed by 14- to 16-year-olds, such as murder, arson, grievous bodily harm, robbery, or behaviour that seriously undermines social order. Below that age young people are considered to be immature physically and psychologically, and not to have enough experience and knowledge to enable them to foresee the possible harmful consequences of their behaviour. Thus decisions about criminal responsibility for those with a mental illness are related to equating behavioural responsibility with that of legal minors (Beijing Medical University, 1986). Two criteria are used. First, the offender should be suffering from an acute, chronic or temporary mental illness. Second, this mental illness must be of such severity that the patient loses the capacity to distinguish right from wrong or to control his or her behaviour. Both criteria must be met simultaneously and both are equally important. Similarity to the McNaughten rules (Prins, 1980, p. 18) is clear:

> "It must be clearly proved that, at the time of the committing of the act, the party accused was labouring under such a defect of reason, from disease of the mind, as not to know the nature and quality of the act he was doing; or if he did know it, that he did not know what he was doing was wrong."

Some authors on this topic (Beijing Medical University, 1986; Zhang Hu, 1987) are familiar with the McNaughten rules but there is no statement that the Chinese system is based on them.

Diminished responsibility

While the 'not guilty by reason of insanity' verdict is relatively rare in the UK (Prins, 1980; Chiswick, 1988) it is the logical consequence of being judged to have no responsibility in China, and is therefore the rule rather than the exception for mentally ill offenders. Officially, Chinese law only recognises an either/or position with regard to criminal responsibility, but in practice, partial or diminished responsibility is also accepted in Chinese courts (Zhang Hu, 1987). Unlike the UK, China applies the concept of diminished responsibility to a variety of offences rather than just to murder.

Yu Dejiang (1987) argues that having a mental illness does not necessarily mean that the offender should escape responsibility for the crime. He suggests that if the offender knows that he has a psychotic illness, if he can objectively criticise his own psychotic symptoms, and if he knows that his psychosis affects his future, his family and society generally, then he can be judged to have sufficient self-awareness to tell the difference between right and wrong and to have controlled his behaviour. Thus he should be dealt with as an ordinary criminal.

There is extensive discussion (Beijing Medical University, 1986; Guo Jingyuan, 1987) as to which mental illnesses should be considered to affect criminal responsibility. The general consensus is that someone in the grip of an acute psychotic episode should be considered to have no criminal responsibility. A patient who is clearly in remission should be judged to have partial or diminished responsibility, based on individual circumstances. The very severely mentally retarded would normally be considered to have no responsibility while those with less retardation would be more likely to be judged as having partial responsibility. People with organic brain damage, for instance caused by arteriosclerosis or Alzheimer's disease, would probably be considered to be able to exercise partial responsibility but the decision would be based on the circumstances of their case, and the severity of their condition. Generally, people suffering from neurosis or personality disorder are to be treated as normal offenders. Zhang Hu (1987) comments on the paradox of the anti-psychiatry movement in the West that favours treating psychiatrically ill offenders as ordinary criminals, "which would lead to the penalising of psychotics when they commit crimes".

What reasons are put forward to justify treating those with a mental illness differently from other accused persons under the law? Guo Jingyuan (1987, p. 153) summarises them:

> "A mentally ill person is not able to assess or control his own behaviour which leads to self-destructive or other destructive behaviour. This is against the requirements of law and society concerning individual's behaviour and will seriously destroy public peace and order, causing damage and loss to society, family and individuals. But from the point of law and medicine we should give more understanding towards criminal acts committed by mental patients and not judge or punish them by ordinary legal standards. The reasons for this are as follows. First, the behaviour of the mental person is a sign of their illness and they cannot control it. Second, people in society should be more understanding to mental patients and show them humanitarian concern. Third, we should give custodial and enforced treatment to the patient. Fourth, punishing a mental patient cannot produce positive results and will cause negative consequences, making their illness worse. Therefore, the law should treat mental patients differently when they have committed crimes."

What should happen if the person is clearly psychotic, and yet the psychosis does not appear to be related to the crime, is controversial (Jia Yicheng, 1983; Zhang Hu, 1986). Some Chinese psychiatrists say that if a direct connection between the crime and the illness cannot be shown, then the person should be treated as an ordinary criminal; others say that the very fact of having a mental illness should mean giving serious consideration to permitting partial responsibility.

The appraisal process

Each provincial or city level Procurator's Department must formally appoint an Assessment Committee on Forensic Psychiatry

(Wu Jiasheng, 1985). The committee should consist of doctors with psychiatric experience, preferably in forensic psychiatry. Their purpose is to conduct a psychiatric examination, and an investigation to determine a person's level of criminal responsibility. This work is mostly done on an out-patient basis. It is not clear from the available information whether most cases would be on remand in jail, or on some form of bail at home.

A request for appraisal may be made by various people at various stages in the legal process. According to Article 75 of the *Criminal Procedure Law of the People's Republic of China* (1979), neither the victim nor the accused may refuse to be physically examined. Zhang & Shi (1987) report research carried out in Hangzhou. Of appraisal requests, 53.4% were made because public security officials detected mental abnormalities in criminals before or during the trial. Only 2.4% of requests were made because offenders showed abnormalities during their imprisonment; 10.5% of requests originated from the families of the accused, which the author suggests shows faith in the judicial system; and 32.9% of requests were made because the accused was known to have been suffering from a mental illness before committing the crime.

In this sample, 46.3% of those appraised were considered to have full criminal responsibility, 29% partial criminal responsibility, and 24% no criminal responsibility.

Appraisal may also be requested to be made of victims. In Zhang's research, all such cases occurred where the victim was the subject of rape or attempted rape and suspected to be mentally retarded.

The appraisal is a group process by two or three panel members. The panel between them is expected to interview the accused, their family, the *danwei*, and anyone else who may be considered to have useful information, as well as examining all relevant documents pertaining to the accusation and trial. At Anding hospital in Beijing I was told that it is usual for the patient to spend about four hours in the forensic assessment unit, during which time he or she will be interviewed and given various tests including an EEG, the Weschler Intelligence Test, the Eysenck Personality Inventory and the MMPI.

The law requires that the accused be informed of the conclusion of the report, which should state clearly whether the appraised should take criminal responsibility, has the ability to understand the proceedings, or is feigning illness (Article 90, *Criminal Procedure Law of the People's Republic of China*, 1979). Article 90 also states that the person being appraised may request a new or supplementary report, presumably if they think the first one is biased or inaccurate in some way. The report is not legally binding. It is submitted to the court and they may or may not choose to accept its recommendations. Zhang & Shi (1987) found that the conclusions of their written reports formed the basis of the court's decision in 91% of cases.

Zhang & Shi talk about 210 cases being referred to their department for an appraisal, but producing only 121 written reports. This is despite the fact that the law requires written reports signed by the appraisers in all cases (Article 89, *Criminal Procedure Law of the People's Republic of China*, 1979). An appraisal can also, apparently, take place in the court (Beijing Medical University, 1986). It seems likely that there are major variations in standards of practice, presumably according to availability of resources and accepted practices from area to area.

Differences of opinion

It is clear from the available literature that the appraisal doctors disagree with each other sometimes. When doctors on the panel disagree they are permitted to submit separate reports, and the court may choose the one that they wish (Beijing Medical University, 1986). It is also said that if the family or the *danwei* (workunit) are not satisfied with the way that the appraisal has been conducted, they are at liberty to request a second opinion. How many of them have the courage or resources to do this is not known.

More serious clashes of opinion occur, best exemplified by an attempted murder case described by Guan Xin (1988). It concerned a slightly physically handicapped man who formed an unreciprocated attachment to a young woman. He went to her house one night and stabbed her and then himself. Both recovered. The defender of the accused requested a psychiatric appraisal. The appraisal report concluded that the accused was suffering from paranoid schizophrenia. The court refused to accept this, saying that:

> "It would not be objective if we said that the accused is deluded by love, just from his love for the victim, and has a delusion of jealousy, just from the fact that the victim has told the accused about her boyfriend. Similar situations happen to many people in real life. Does this mean that all of them are suffering from paranoid schizophrenia?" (Guan Xin, 1988, p. 38)

So, the court asked for another assessment from a different hospital. This reached the exactly opposite conclusion from the first: that the accused should bear full responsibility as he was not suffering from a mental illness. As a result this was adjudged a 'difficult' case, and was suspended for 18 months. It seems that it was then referred to the provincial high court where the judges questioned the accused and his family, interviewed the victim, made investigations at the place where the offence occurred, and eventually concluded that they supported the findings of the second report.

This case clearly indicates that the court is not obliged to accept medical opinion if it does not concur with its own. While one interpretation is that the court is able to seek several opinions, until it finds one which agrees with the already established opinion of the court, this view may be too cynical. In the case outlined, much effort seems to have been taken to be fair to the accused, and not to reach a hasty decision that was not backed by strong medical opinion. It is noticeable that the psychiatric opinions sought came from institutions of increasingly higher reputation.

Crime categories

Information on the type of crimes for which appraisals are requested is scarce and incomplete, as is that concerning the frequency of each kind of diagnostic category. In the sample of Zhang & Shi (1987) sexual crimes were the most frequent (35%), mostly involving rape or attempted rape. It is not wholly clear from their figures, but it seems that the majority of victims and perpetrators were mentally handicapped. One wonders how 'rape' is being defined in these circumstances, and to what extent the term is being used to describe consensual intercourse between people who are not deemed socially entitled to it.

Zhang & Shi's second category is a ragbag of murder, assault, theft, fraud, arson, framing others, antisocial and anti-political speeches and deeds. Of these cases, in 1977, 54% of crimes by those being appraised concerned anti-political actions. Now the figure has dropped to 6.7%, which "shows that there is internal stability and unity in China". There is no discussion of whether this is an absolute drop in numbers due to a decrease in that kind of crime, or whether the officials of the Public Security Bureau now only take notice of such behaviour if it is very extreme.

Zhang & Shi claim that in their survey, 30.9% of those appraised were diagnosed as mentally retarded, 23.3% were suffering from schizophrenia, and 7.2% suffered from a personality disorder. Other studies found that the majority were suffering from schizophrenia. For example, a major study by Li Congpei (1987) of 865 cases of psychiatric appraisal, found that 45% were diagnosed with schizophrenia. Of those, 79% were males, of whom 75% were between the ages of 21 and 40. Among the victims of the people suffering from schizophrenia, 51% were relatives. The appraisers of the offenders with schizophrenia judged that 97.5% were not responsible for their actions.

Ability to stand trial

The Beijing Medical University text (1986) points out that the capacity to stand trial needs to be distinguished from the ability to accept criminal responsibility. The latter refers to the accused's state of mind at the time of the crime. The former is only concerned with whether the accused is able to properly take part in court proceedings, by being able to understand the nature and process of the trial, and being able to cooperate with his or her lawyer. In some cases the accused may be exempted on both counts. If the accused is judged not to be capable of taking part in the trial, then he or she is to be 'convinced to take treatment', and the trial will be postponed until the person is fit to stand. While not ideal, this has some advantages in comparison with the British system, where someone who is considered unfit to plead may be consigned to a secure hospital, and is effectively given an indeterminate sentence without having been found guilty or had the chance to present a defence to the court. In the UK, such cases are apparently rarely brought back to court (Prins, 1980; Chiswick, 1988).

Offenders with a mental illness

The original articles that have been drawn on so far discuss the details of criminal responsibility in repetitive detail. However, they are noticeably silent on what happens to those who are found to be suffering from a mental illness, and who are consequently considered to have no responsibility and are therefore not guilty. Are they permitted to return to their families under strict supervision? Are they hospitalised in ordinary institutions? And if so, how is the length of their stay determined? Are there special institutions for severely mentally ill offenders, even if they have not been sentenced?

Two pieces of legislation give some guidance on this matter. The first is Article 37 of the *Act of the People's Republic of China for Reform Through Labour*, promulgated in 1954. As quoted in Leng & Chiu (1985, p. 253):

"A health examination shall be given to offenders who are committed to custody. Except for counter-revolutionary offenders whose criminal acts are major, commitment to custody shall not be permitted in any one of the following circumstances (i) mental illness or acute or malignant contagious disease...(ii) offenders who under the preceding items may not be committed to custody shall, after the organ that originally ordered their commitment to custody has considered the situation, be sent to a hospital, turned over to a guardian, or put in another appropriate place."

Regulations of the People's Republic of China on Administrative Penalties for Public Security, 1986, Article 10 states:

"A mentally disordered person who violates the administration of public security at a time when he is unable to account for or control his conduct, shall not be penalised, but his guardian shall be instructed to keep a close watch on him and subject him to medical treatment." (*China Law Year Book,* 1987)

Shanghai regulations

Shanghai has produced its own 'mini' version of a mental health law, called the *Regulations of the Shanghai Municipality on Guardianship, Treatment and Handling of Mental Patients Stirring Up Trouble and Causing Disasters* (*China Law Year Book,* 1987). This was adopted at the 23rd session of the Standing Committee of the Eighth People's Congress of Shanghai Municipality in August 1986. Article 8 defines 'stirring up trouble' as:
  (a) Committing assault or doing violence causing injury to others
  (b) Insulting women
  (c) Damaging public or private property
  (d) Impeding the safety of communication
  (e) Other acts disrupting public order or hampering public security.
Article 11 authorises officers of the Public Security Bureau to remove by force to hospital for treatment someone whom they think is suffering from a mental illness, and who is stirring up trouble, with or without the relatives' permission. The same article says that the patient must be examined on arrival at the hospital by two doctors, one of whom must be on the level of physician-in-charge. If this doctor decides that the person is not suffering from a mental illness, then the Public Security staff will "deal with him according to the law".

Other articles deal with relatives who wish to discharge a patient without the permission of the hospital authorities; they are not allowed to do so. Under these regulations, if treatment is completed but patients' families are unwilling to accept them back, the Public Security Bureau are authorised to escort patients from the hospital and deliver them to their relatives, whether they are willing or not.

The category of 'causing disasters' is more serious and includes homicide, rape, arson, causing explosions, robbery, poison and other acts seriously endangering public security. These people must be examined by the expert appraisal panel. These patients need not only the approval of the hospital but also of the Public Security Bureau before they can be discharged.

There are at least two areas in which these regulations are different from common practice in China. First, they permit the wishes of the relatives to be overruled, albeit in cases which are considered to be serious. Second, for both categories of patient, the regulations (Articles 11 and 14) say that the expert appraisal panel may be used as an appeal body by patients, relatives or victims not satisfied with the diagnosis or hospitalisation.

While these various laws and regulations give some idea of what happens in theory, and are coherent with the general notion of clemency towards those with a mental illness found in Chinese law, they offer no clue as to what happens in practice.

Practical applications

Reading through files at the Municipal Hospital, it rapidly became clear that there were people there who had technically broken the law, been arrested or 'picked up' by the Public Security Bureau, and taken straight to hospital. There seems to have been agreement between the Public Security Bureau representative, and the family or street organisation responsible for the patient, that their behaviour was so clearly crazy that arranging an admission to a hospital was obviously the most sensible course of action. For instance, one female patient with a history of criminal damage (not specified), scolding and hitting people in the street, and stripping naked in public and standing in the road stopping traffic, was arrested and brought to the hospital, with her family's approval.

Another male patient disturbed traffic, destroyed his own clothes, attacked his father with an axe, assaulted women on the street, set fire to his house, and "affected social security with very, very, bad consequences". He was admitted through the Public Security

Bureau at the request of his family. Similarly, a male patient, with no family to support him, was admitted at the request of his street organisation after he hit people and broke windows and the glass front door of a hotel, and was deemed to "have seriously affected social security". Such decisions are in line with the provisions of Article 37 of the 1954 *Law of the People's Republic of China for Reform Through Labour*. Presumably, such a disposal would be more acceptable to relatives than a public trial and possible imprisonment.

The most outstanding example of these laws at work that I have personally come across concerned a 15-year-old young man I interviewed soon after his admission to a hospital in Hubei province. After a disastrous love affair with his young, female, class teacher, he had stolen dynamite from a local quarry, wrapped it up so it looked like a gift, and given it to her in the hopes that it would blow her up. The Public Security Bureau, on the grounds that this behaviour was so outrageous that the boy must be crazy, offered his father two alternatives: a court appearance and an inevitable jail sentence, or immediate admission to psychiatric hospital. The father chose hospital as the lesser of the two evils.

Prins (1980) points out that police in England will often unofficially screen out petty offenders whom they consider to be mentally disturbed, if other arrangements they consider more suitable than a trial can be made. Section 136 of the Mental Health Amendment Act (1983) permits the police to remove from a public place to a place of safety someone whom they consider to be mentally disordered. Often this place will be a psychiatric hospital.

An Cun hospitals

For those who are thought to be seriously psychotic, who have committed a dangerous offence, but who have been found to have nil responsibility, 'guardianship' may still have to be provided at the discretion of the court (Zhang Iiu, 1987). There are special hospitals run by the Public Security Bureau for people who have been found to have partial responsibility, and for those who are deemed to be very dangerous, even though they have been judged to have nil responsibility. In theory, every province and the three municipalities directly under the Central Government (Shanghai, Beijing and Tianjin) should have such a hospital.

Wu Jiasheng (1985) writes in some detail of these "treatment and management institutes for mentally ill offenders". Mentally ill offenders who require custodial treatment need a special case report by the local Public Security unit. This, together with the forensic psychiatry appraisal report, has to be evaluated and approved at the provincial or city level by the Public Security Bureau. Offenders should be given modern treatment for their illness, and once they have become stable they should be given appropriate cultural education and assigned some light labour work, so as to help them recover their ability to live in the community. Once the patients are definitely cured, they can go back to their work units, or to the care of their neighbourhood committees. Wu also implies that the offender–patient will continue to receive money from his work unit during his stay, "according to the Labour Ordinance".

In discussion with a doctor at Anding Hospital, Beijing, who worked in the forensic assessment unit there, I was told that if a patient referred by the Public Security Bureau is found not to be able to bear criminal responsibility, then the Public Security Bureau is responsible for his disposal. They might let him return to his family, or they might decide to admit him to one of the special psychiatric hospitals. All of these Public Security Bureau hospitals are known by the name 'An Cun', for example Beijing An Cun Hospital.

It is unlikely that the police would return someone who had committed a felony to his family, but they would be more inclined to do so if the offence was classified as a misdemeanour. Once admitted to such a hospital, the offender who has committed a more serious crime is likely to spend some years there. Someone with a less serious offence may be discharged once his mental state is considered to be stable.

Doctors working at An Cun hospitals will make a recommendation for discharge to the hospital leaders, who are Public Security Bureau officials and who take the final responsibility. The leaders take into account both the patient's mental state and the family's willingness to look after the patient, but apparently most of all the current 'community atmosphere'. Patients are less likely to be released during times of unrest, or during an important event, such as the Asian Games.

Offenders who are found to have diminished responsibility may also be admitted to an An Cun hospital, and in practice they are treated no differently from those found to have no responsibility. There is also a psychiatric prison hospital in a county just outside Beijing; prisoners who become mentally ill in prison go there. Not all patients who offend are sent to an An Cun hospital. Some of them may be admitted to an ordinary hospital, if the hospital is willing to take them. This is not surprising when one considers that, in China, all hospitals are extremely security conscious.

Time scales

Within the prison and special hospital system in the UK, both staff and offenders are very aware of the concept 'time for the crime' (Peay, 1989). My own experience of working in Broadmoor led to the observation that there is a reluctance to discharge someone from a special hospital, even when the illness is under control, unless he has served as much time as would have been likely had he received a prison term. Mental illness is not an issue in deciding guilt or innocence in the UK, but rather disposal once guilt has been established. Within the Chinese system, an offender who is mentally ill is technically not guilty of the crime because of his insanity. Thus, while in effect 'sentenced' to hospital (despite being innocent of the crime), he may spend less time there than he would have spent in prison. Certainly, the two doctors to whom I spoke on the subject did not emphasise the question of parity.

Sun Junwen (1984) describes six cases of patients with schizophrenia who, while in Zhejiang Provincial Psychiatric Hospital, killed fellow patients. Three of these patients were discharged: one within three and a half years of the murder; one within one year; and one within one month. All were described as responding well to treatment.

A case example may serve to illustrate some of the intricacies involved (Beijing Medical University, 1986). In 1967 a man called Wang, with others, was implicated in a murder which was assumed to have happened after the supposed victim disappeared. Wang was asked to sign a letter of confession which he did, without the proper investigations being carried out. It is suggested in the article that this was at the height of the Cultural Revolution and political grudges were involved. Wang was a model prisoner, and although those convicted with him appealed against their sentences, he never did. No mental abnormality was detected until he had been in prison for a year or so, and he requested to join the Communist Party. He claimed that the party had appointed him its central investigator, number 808.

The authorities did nothing at that time, but three years later, when he claimed that the Party had commanded him, through a "highly confidential television set", to commit the murder, they decided that it was time to have him appraised. The investigating psychiatrists discovered an encapsulated delusional system involving Wang's relationship, as he perceived it, with the Party, and his belief that his behaviour was completely controlled by television and an electronic man inside his body. They decided that his confession was part of his delusional system, and that he had never been involved in a murder. They recommended that he should be exempted from criminal responsibility. The various government departments involved ruled that the case had been wrongly decided, and reinstated Wang's reputation. They also provided him with work and treatment.

The civil law

Within civil law, there is an idea that corresponds to that of criminal responsibility, the ability to 'act' which is based on whether or not a patient is able to understand his civil rights and obligations and to carry them out (Guo Jingyuan, 1987). This largely affects marriage, entering into contracts and making a will. Once again the analogy is that of legal minors. Children below the age of ten are considered not to be able to enter into any legal agreement (Article 12, *General Principles of the Civil Law of China*, 1986). Their rights and obligations are exercised on their behalf by their parents, who are also expected to protect their interests. Children between the ages of 10 and 18 are considered to be partially responsible in this respect (Articles 11 and 12, *General Principles of the Civil Law of China*, 1986). A "person with no capacity to engage in litigation" shall be represented in action by guardians who will be statutory agents. If they try to shift the burden of responsibility from one to the other, the court shall appoint one of them to represent the principal in the action. Lawyers, close relatives of the party concerned, persons recommended by relevant social organisations or by the work units of the person concerned and any other citizens approved by the People's Court, may be appointed guardian *ad litem* (Article 57, *Civil Procedure Law of the People's Republic of China*, 1991).

Relatives or other interested parties may apply to the court to have a citizen determined as having no capacity for civil acts (or limited capacity). The court may, when necessary, carry out an expert evaluation and if the health of such an individual permits, the court shall solicit their opinion. People who have been deemed incompetent may take their case back to the court at a later stage and if they are able to demonstrate that their situation has changed, civil capacity can be restored (Articles 170–173, *Civil Procedure Law of the People's Republic of China*, 1991).

The court is empowered to appoint a guardian, usually a relative, who will have similar rights over the patient to those a parent has over a child. If no relative is willing or able to act, then this role is expected to be taken up by the *danwei*, neighbourhood or village committee, or local Civil Affairs Bureau, as appropriate (Article 17, *General Principles of the Civil Law of China*, 1986).

The guardian becomes responsible in law for the actions of the person with a mental illness. Thus, if that person causes damage and compensation has to be paid, the guardian must pay it, unless the guardian can prove to the court's satisfaction that the person is beyond his control (Article 8, *Regulations of the People's Republic of China on Administrative Penalties for Public Security*, 1986). In turn, if the guardian through handling his charge's property makes a loss, the guardian is responsible for repaying the money or goods so lost (Article 18, *General Principles of the Civil Law of the People's Republic of China*, 1986). Any person who 'shares interests' with the mental patient may apply to the People's Court for a declaration that the mental patient is incompetent for civil conduct, or is limited in such conduct (Article 19, *General Principles of the Civil Law of the People's Republic of China*, 1986). The removal of civil responsibility would only be considered in cases where the mental impairment seems to be permanent and of long-standing duration. It would not be considered in cases of temporary or intermittent disturbance of sanity (Beijing Medical University, 1986).

The following examples are given. If a party to a marriage suspects that the other party has a mental illness and he or she wants to nullify the marriage, it is possible to apply to have the partner's psychiatric state appraised by the court. Wills may also be challenged on the grounds that the deceased was not in his right mind at the time of drawing up the will. In this case, the appraisal procedure must be carried out using secondary sources of evidence. A contract is invalid if one of the parties to it is found not to have been able to exercise civil competence at the time of the contract. If the person lacking civil competence suffers a loss as a consequence, the other party has to pay compensation. Parents who suffer from a severe mental illness and lack civil responsibility, may lose their parental rights. Nathan (1986*a*) says that those with a mental illness are not permitted to vote. Article 37 of the *Criminal Procedure Law of the People's Republic of China*, 1979, forbids people who have physical or mental handicaps, who are too young to know right from wrong, or who cannot adequately express their own will, from being witnesses in court.

A case illustrating how this legal provision might be used is given (Beijing Medical University, 1986). On several occasions a cadre in a rural area wandered away from home, staying out all night and causing a search to be made for him. He was found dishevelled and apparently having been faecally incontinent. On the last occasion he stayed away for ten days, eventually returning by himself exhausted. On all three occasions he was unable to remember what had happened. People "began to suspect that he was abnormal" and he was sent for a psychiatric appraisal. Although normal in every respect on a verbal examination he was given an EEG and found to have abnormal brainwaves associated with epilepsy. On these grounds he was ruled to have neither criminal responsibility nor civil competence.

Involuntary commitment

However, losing one's civil competence does not necessarily imply involuntary commitment to psychiatric hospital. It has been widely reported by Western observers either that there are no compulsory admissions to psychiatric hospitals in China or that they are very rare. Visher &Visher (1979) state that compulsory admission of patients does not occur in China except in criminal cases. Bloomingdale (1980, p. 23) asserts that:

> "Forensic psychiatry does not exist in the People's Republic of China....Chinese psychiatrists were puzzled about Western insanity laws. In China the issue of legal sanity is not raised."

Breger (1984, p. 130) claims that:

> "When hospitalisation is deemed necessary, patients are admitted voluntarily, invariably persuaded and not forced to enter hospital. We saw no evidence of a civil commitment process."

Breger is correct when he says that no process of civil commitment exists, but is wrong to assume that there are no compulsory admissions. It is perhaps difficult for a Western observer, steeped in the belief that it is necessary to protect individual freedom, to perceive that it is perfectly possible to put someone in hospital without their permission, and with no legal protection at all.

The Chinese view is more concerned with the patient's right to receive treatment, and doubtless with society's need to be protected. It was clear from the files at the Municipal Hospital that many people were brought to hospital against their will. One was admitted in chains by the Public Security Bureau. Another was tricked by her family into believing that they were all going on a picnic to the country. In Shashi psychiatric hospital, one patient from the rural area was brought to the hospital by his family trussed up as thoroughly as a turkey ready for the oven. The only action still available to him was to spit.

It is not the individual who is consulted about admission, but the family. If the family agrees to it, then the patient is admitted. If the family disagrees then the patient stays outside until such time as the bizarre behaviour comes to the attention of the Public Security Bureau (if it ever does), or the family reaches a stage when it can no longer cope and changes its mind. Some of the cases cited earlier in the chapter are a testimony to the level of disturbed behaviour some families are willing to tolerate before taking action.

Marriage and mental illness

The 1950 Marriage Law forbade those with learning difficulties, but not those with a mental illness, from getting married. Over the years, attitudes changed somewhat, so that marriage was seen as a right whose benefits those with a learning disability should be able to enjoy. On the other hand, bearing children was a privilege and should be strictly controlled. The situation of people with a mental illness has changed with the new Marriage Law of 1980. Article 6(b) states:

> "Marriage is not permitted in the following circumstances....Where one party is suffering from leprosy, a cure not having been affected, or from any other disease which is regarded by medical science as rendering a person unfit for marriage."

Clearly, this leaves a great deal of space for individual interpretation by different provinces and municipalities. Palmer (1987) reports a case of a 35-year-old woman who applied to the court for a divorce after six years of marriage to a man who habitually beat and abused her, even following her to her workplace to do so. He was diagnosed as suffering from schizophrenia and she applied to the court for a divorce on the grounds that he was suffering from an illness "regarded by medical science as rendering a person unfit for marriage". The court refused her request, instead instructing her to "go away and perform to the fullest extent the duties of a wife". It appeared that her father-in-law had exerted influence with the court because he did not want to have the responsibility of looking after his mentally deranged son and was afraid of losing custody of his grandson.

An authoritative commentary on the Marriage Law (Ren Guojun, 1988) confirms that the law is not clear and that the relevant judicial and legislative organs have not yet issued any interpretations. Based on judicial practice, the two most important illnesses covered by Article 6(b) are severe mental illness (he mentions schizophrenia and manic-depression specifically), and learning disability. Three reasons are given as to why schizophrenia and manic-depression constitute an obstacle to marriage.

(a) Both illnesses are contracted during youth
(b) Patients suffering from schizophrenia in particular are unable to take legal responsibility, suffer from a lack of self-control, and lack the ability to exercise civil competence. Consequently, they are unable to exercise marital or parental responsibilities
(c) Both schizophrenia and manic-depression are hereditable diseases. Thus there is a danger of transmitting them to descendants, and the risk of spreading the disease through the population is very great. Ren emphasises that this is the most basic reason.

Birth control

There is no doubt at all that Chinese psychiatrists are very concerned about the hereditability of schizophrenia (Fang Yongzhang, 1982; Liu Xiehe, 1983; Xun Minlai, 1986). Some see it as a justification for restricting marriage and childbirth. In such a populous nation, it is hardly surprising that measures taken to control the birth rate are more stringent than are considered appropriate in the West. Both Fang Yongzhang (1982) and Xun Minlai (1986) are concerned with the higher birth rate among women diagnosed as suffering from schizophrenia among whom, for a variety of reasons, birth control acceptance is not high. One reason is that birth control workers are afraid of them, and reluctant to approach them or 'mobilise' them in the face of resistance, in the same way they would other members of the population. Both Xun and Fang advocate using the law to restrict marriage and childbirth for people suffering from schizophrenia, and frankly advocate a policy of eugenics and compulsory sterilisation. Xun's research involved a population of 250 men and women with schizophrenia who were sterilised in the Xiang Tan Psychiatric Hospital in Hunan Province, between 1972 and 1983. What is not made clear is whether these sterilisations were voluntary or not. Likewise, Fang mentions that 22% of his sample of people with schizophrenia were sterilised.

In 1986, the Ministry of Public Health and the Ministry of Civil Affairs issued a *Circular Concerning Premarital Medical Check-ups* (Zhi Ming, 1991). The circular stipulates that the parties concerned can only complete the marriage registration formalities after they have undergone a medical examination, although there is the proviso that "since conditions vary from place to place, no fixed time for implementing the circular has been laid down". The circular has three categories affecting marriage and childbirth. Marriage is prohibited between close relatives and between people who have very low intelligence. Marriage is to be postponed when one or both parties are suffering from schizo-phrenia, manic-depression, or other types of psychoses. Marriage is permitted but childbirth forbidden:

"...where either party whose inherited disease, such as schizophrenia, manic-depressive psychosis, or other types of psychoses, as well as congenital heart disease is in a stable condition" (Zhi Ming, 1991, p. 18).

In 1989, 113 000 people underwent the premarital examination and 1.4% of them suffered from problems affecting their proposed marriage. Thirteen were prohibited from marriage and 1479 had to delay their marriage. The aim of this policy is quite clear:

"With the rapid development of eugenics, scientific research work into eugenics and healthier births broke new ground, and health care work in urban and rural areas greatly improved, thereby enabling eugenics to guide marriage and childbirth." (Zhi Ming, 1991, p. 18)

Thus, although the Marriage Law is very nonspecific, it does appear that there are regulations restricting marriage and childbirth for people suffering from mental illness in China. What is completely unknown is how rigorously and universally these are enforced, and how many people are persuaded or forced to accept sterilisation.

In December 1993, the official Xinhua news agency announced that a Draft Law on Eugenics and Health Protection was under consideration (*Far East Economic Review*, 13 January 1994, p. 22). This draft law aims to prevent new births of inferior quality people and heighten the standards of the whole population. It promotes sterilisation, abortions or celibacy for people with hereditary, venereal or reproductive ailments, severe psychoses or contagious diseases. The announcement of the draft law caused little excitement in the Chinese press, but the reaction overseas was much more vigorous. The English name was then changed to the 'Maternal and Infant Health Care Law', but remained the same in Chinese. The law was promulgated in October 1994 and came into effect in June 1995. Its effects and the willingness of doctors and psychiatrists to put it into practice cannot be assessed. Such policies are another manifestation of priorities that place the good of the collective higher than the wishes or rights of the individual (Pearson, 1995*b*).

Human rights issues

A definition in the West of human rights would probably be based on international agreements such as the *Universal Declaration of Human Rights*, 1948, the *International Covenant on Civil and Political Rights*, 1966, and the *International Covenant on Economic, Social, and Cultural Rights*, 1966.

It is generally agreed that the question of human or civil rights did not feature in traditional Chinese moral or political philosophy. Hansen (1985) claims that the term 'rights' only entered the Chinese vocabulary in comparatively modern times. Wang Gung Wu (1979) argues that, at least initially, the presence of duties, particularly filial piety and loyalty, also implies the presence of rights. If a son is filial, he has a right to expect a mother to be loving and caring. If a subject is loyal, he has a right to expect the Emperor to be benevolent. However, these duties and implied rights were between unequals, which in turn led to an uneven distribution of both duties and rights. The resulting picture was one of a civilisation where the great majority had only duties, and the only rights were found among the small minority who held power above (Wang Gung Wu, 1979).

Despotism emerged gradually over the centuries, worsening steadily from the Han to the Tang dynasties and more rapidly after the Tang, reaching new heights during the Ming and Qing dynasties. The Confucian moral order contained no belief in the rights of the individual as a limit on any kind of authority be it familial or state. Indeed, Kamenka (1978, p. 8) comments that:

"The Great Code of Punishments of the Qing Dynasty was as complex and sophisticated an administrative document as any European *lex* or *leges* up to even the nineteenth century; but it was a code of punishments, addressed to officials and not to the citizens, providing administrative measures, imposing strict obligations while encouraging *ad hoc* justice and sub-legal settlement."

Tao (1990) made the point that the Chinese way of thinking about the self and about moral agency is in stark contrast to the image of self as a bearer of rights – rather, the collective good and of membership in a society is valued. This was apparent in the approach of the late nineteenth and early twentieth century political reformers in China. They became interested in the question of rights, many of them having been educated overseas, and rights became part of the reformist agenda. However, they largely addressed the question of rights and liberties from the perspective of what would best serve collective goals and when they discussed individual rights it was in terms of how exercising such rights could best strengthen China, for instance, by releasing individual creativity and energy to be put to work solving China's many problems. Such rights were not universal principles but instruments towards a higher goal, that of strengthening China (Wu Wang Gung, 1979).

John C. H. Wu, a jurist responsible among other things for drafting China's 1946 constitution, expressed it this way:

> "Westerners, in struggling for freedom, started from the individual. Now we, in struggling for freedom, started from the group...We wish to save the nation and the race and so we cannot but demand that each individual sacrifices his own freedom in order to preserve the freedom of the group." (quoted in Wang Gung Wu, 1979, p. 29)

A component in modern China's attitude towards human rights is the traditional Marxist distrust and ambivalence towards them. While human rights may have been instrumental in political change they were, at the same time, seen to be statements of the demands of the bourgeoisie, and of the necessary conditions of capitalism to own property and buy and sell freely (Tay, 1978). For Marx, the ideal was not the individual man, but the social man subsumed into a collective unit. Furthermore, at least in their original formulation, human rights were seen as rights of citizens against governments, not a welcome perspective in any autocracy (Minogue, 1978).

Since 1949, China has had four constitutions: in 1954, 1975, 1978 and 1982. The latter was amended in 1988 and again in 1993 by the Eighth People's Congress. Amendments concerned economic rather than political reform, and their adoption has brought the constitution in line with changes in the Communist Party's economic policy (Conner, 1993). It is not necessary to examine the content in detail for the purposes of the present discussion. In many ways, the 1982 Chinese constitution is a model of its kind. It guarantees equality before the law; the right to vote and stand in election; the freedom of speech; of the press; of assembly; of association; of demonstration; religious belief; freedom of correspondence; the right to make complaints against state organs or functionaries. At this point, it is essential to recall Cranston's injunction (1973) to "keep in mind the distinction between what is and what ought to be, between the empirical and the normative".

In none of the constitutions were rights considered to be derived from human personhood. They were received from the state and were not considered to apply to all. Before 1982, distinctions were made between 'the people', who were usually workers and poor peasants, and those with a bad class background like landowners, or those who were considered to oppose the purposes of the state and were dubbed counter-revolutionary. The rights in China's constitution are the rights of citizens, not of persons. Citizenship is not constitutionally guaranteed, so that a person who is not accorded, or is deprived, of citizenship is not promised any rights at all.

Chinese constitution writers had no inhibitions about changing provisions in the constitution quite dramatically to suit altered circumstances. What the state could dispense it could equally well withdraw:

> "Rights are entrusted by society to the individual; society is the source of rights. The individual apart from society has no rights to speak of. Since society bestows rights, at times of necessity it can also remove rights; at least it can limit their scope". (John C. H. Wu, quoted in Nathan, 1986*b*)

Because rights are granted as part of being a member of society they cannot be enforced against society. There is no concept of the individual needing to be protected from the depredations of the state, or that government is other than positive. The state is considered to be the embodiment of the interests of the people who, therefore, cannot have interests that conflict with those of the state (Kent, 1993).

The Chinese constitutions were written as political programmes for the future, and presented as goals to be realised (Kent, 1993). Thus they mentioned rights which, in fact, could not be enjoyed (Nathan, 1986*a*). These constitutions did not form a contract between the governed and the government, embodying sets of reciprocal rights and duties. Their main function was to create a strong state, not to restrict the powers of the state.

In November, 1989 the *Beijing Review* (6 November, 1989) carried an article entitled *Opposing Interference In Other Countries' Internal Affairs Through Human Rights* by Yi Ding. This article denies that there are any universal or abstract human rights. It states that human rights are only those which have been recognised in law by the dominant class of a country; that there are no universal human rights which override the laws of various countries; and that international documents relating to human rights do not supersede the laws of any country.

These views were embodied in a White Paper, *Human Rights In China,* published in 1991. Essentially, this was a riposte to the increasing international pressure that China has come under regarding her record on human rights, particularly since the events in Tiananmen Square in 1989, and their sequelae. China's two basic positions are summed up thus:

"To the people in the developing countries, the most urgent human rights are still the right to subsistence and the right to economic, social and cultural development...China has firmly opposed any country making use of the issue of human rights to sell its own values, ideology, political standards and mode of development and to any country interfering in the internal affairs of other countries on the pretext of human rights, the internal affairs of developing countries in particular and so hurting the sovereignty and dignity of many developing countries...Using the human rights issue for the purpose of imposing the ideology of one country on another is no longer a question of human rights but a manifestation of power politics."

Recent human rights formulations

The West's concern with the universality of human rights has extended more specifically to the rights of those with a mental illness. Statements about their rights, designed to delineate international standards, have been produced by the Minority Rights Group (Heginbotham, 1987); the World Federation of Mental Health (*The Luxor Declaration*) 1989; the United Nations (Daes, 1986) and the World Health Organization (Gostin, 1987*a*).

It has to be said that the concerns embodied in these documents do not reflect priorities in the Chinese situation, where informed consent and legal representation are almost unheard of. A Chinese response might well be that individuals with a mental illness cannot be expected to know what is in their own best interests. If they refuse treatment, it is only another indication of how much they require treatment. If treatment is accepted, it is an indication of a sincere desire to become well. The individual's consent to treatment is simply not an issue in China. Where any thought is given to the matter, it is considered to be a family affair. All that stands between an unwilling patient and a locked ward is the opinion of a relative. Neither in reading Chinese material, nor in discussion with Chinese colleagues, is there any sense that the relatives' interests and those of the patient may clash. None of the financial, emotional or sexual undercurrents that may muddy the clear pool of familial harmony are allowed to disturb the belief that the family always knows and acts in the best interests of its individual members.

Psychiatric hospitals and political detainees

Despite considerable access to both patients and their files, I have found no evidence that sane people are being detained for political offences in the hospitals with which I am familiar. When the direct question has been put as to whether this happens in China, the response tends to be that there is no need. There are other ways of dealing with political dissidents that have already been described and that do not require the inappropriate use of an expensive hospital bed (Pearson, 1992b).

Other Westerners have also asked about this issue. Bloomingdale (1980) was told that political dissidents were sent to May 7th Schools for intensive 'ideological education', not to psychiatric hospitals. Brown (1980) states that 'bad elements' are not sent to psychiatric hospitals. Achtenberg (1983, p. 373) was informed that "mental hospital beds were too scarce to be used for political dissidents". Kleinman (1988) "saw little in the way of conflict and abuse".

There are undoubtedly people in psychiatric hospitals whose breakdowns have been precipitated by political events, or persecution for political reasons, but that is a different matter. There is also a grey area where someone does something that is considered to be so foolhardy by others that the only explanation must be that the perpetrator is mad. For instance, Wu Xinchen (1983) looked at the types of schizophrenia found in a sample of people who had been appraised, and the kinds of crimes they had committed. The most frequent crime was murder or attempted murder (51.9%), but the second most frequent crime was anti-social and anti-political actions (33.6%). Wu says that:

"Most of these cases involve purposeless scribblings, or sticking up posters which carried anti-revolutionary and absurd sayings, or chanting anti-revolutionary slogans." (1983, p. 339)

This kind of crime tended to be committed by those he describes as "deteriorated schizophrenics", or suffering from "delusions of exaggeration". The Beijing Medical University text (1986) gives as an example of a lack of self-control or judgement that typifies crimes committed by people with schizophrenia, "sending anti-revolutionary letters signed in their own name, or even giving their home address and the department they work for". However, the human rights organisation, Human Rights Watch (Asia), has expressed increasing concern that the An Cun system of hospitals (run by the Ministry of Public Security) may well be used to incarcerate political dissidents. Ironically, a recent article by Nathan (1994) reports that in 1964 the Chinese Communist Party criticised the Russian authorities for using the psychiatric system to control those with " the courage to speak out, resist, or fight" (p. 625).

Conclusions

The tradition of jural law, including the separation between the judiciary and the state, has never been strong in China. Societal law, based as it is on moral precepts, lends itself to domination by a class of people or organisation. At one stage, it was the Mandarin class. Now, it is the Party. Within this context, it is not always possible to know what the law is, or whether or not a particular action transgresses it. The Public Security Bureau are given wide-ranging powers to coerce socially and politically compliant behaviour, including detention without the formality of a court appearance.

There are no legal protections for those with a mental illness against involuntary detention or compulsory treatment. In a society where the rule of law is not well established it cannot be said that they are being singled out in this respect. There are few safeguards for anyone in China.

By it's standards, China might be said to have a tradition of showing clemency to people with a mental illness, as far as offending against the law is concerned. Traditionally, they were subject to lesser punishments, and currently, for other than the most serious offences, they are more likely to go to hospital than prison.

The civil law permits a form of guardianship for those people severely incapacitated by mental illness, and who are thought to be incapable of exercising their rights and responsibilities in law. No figures seem to be available to indicate how common this procedure is. The position regarding marriage is not entirely clear. While the Marriage Law does not specifically limit the rights of those suffering from mental illness to marry and have children, supplementary regulations issued by the Ministries of Public Health and Civil Affairs do. Once more, it is impossible to know with any accuracy how consistently, and with what severity, these regulations are carried out. Some psychiatrists are very concerned about the spread of schizophrenia in the population and openly advocate a policy of eugenics.

Legislation that concerns those with a mental illness often represents an uneasy balance between the rights of the individual to freedom and the rights of community to protection. The position in China over the centuries reflects a concern with public order and security that dominates any consideration for the well-being of the individual.

There is, as yet, no firm evidence that Chinese psychiatrists have systematically perverted psychiatry for the purposes of incarceration of dissidents, as has been the case in Russia (Medvedev & Medvedev, 1971; Cohen,1989). However, concern has been expressed that the An Cun system is being misused in this way. There does not seem to be the widespread use of a category of disorder that corresponds to that of 'sluggish schizophrenia' in the old USSR (Wing, 1978).

It is obvious that, while the international community is prepared to publicly criticise Russia, South Africa, the UK, Cuba, Japan and Greece concerning aspects of psychiatric care, China remains largely free of this sort of scrutiny, despite the fact that many of her psychiatric practices are unsatisfactory by international standards.

3   Health and social policy

"Citizens of the People's Republic of China have the right to material assistance from the state and society when they are old, ill or disabled. The state develops the social insurance, social relief and medical and health services that are required to enable citizens to enjoy this right. The state and society ensure the livelihood of disabled members of the armed forces, provide pensions to the families of martyrs and give preferential treatment to the families of military personnel. The state and society help make arrangements for the work, livelihood and education of the blind, deaf-mutes and other handicapped citizens". (Article 45 of the *Constitution of the People's Republic of China*, 1982)

China is capable of launching satellites and building Silkworm missiles yet rice is still planted and tended by hand, and a water buffalo, and perhaps a donkey, are the closest many farms come to mechanisation. It is a society of marked contrasts between rural and urban, modern and traditional, ideological and practical. While Article 45 of the Constitution expresses what the government would like to happen, it has not yet overcome the enormous logistical difficulties involved in ensuring health and welfare for almost 1.2 billion people.

The structure of welfare

There has been a tendency in Western countries to define welfare as something that the state provides for its needy and vulnerable citizens. This has obscured the fundamental reality that the majority of care is provided via family members. Most often this care is offered by unpaid women – mothers, daughters and wives. As it is unpaid, it has also been unrecognised (Perring *et al*, 1990). The concept of the 'welfare mix', developed to take account of the various sources of welfare in any society, provides a framework within which welfare provision in most societies may be analysed (Higgins, 1981; Pinker, 1985; Rose & Shiratori, 1986). In addition to the family, these sources might include the state, employers, trade unions, commercial and non-governmental organisations (Higgins, 1986).

The 'welfare mix' in China may be conceptualised as three concentric circles with the family at the centre, the collective (which may be represented by the *danwei* or by the neighbourhood/ street organisation) in the next ring, and then the state as the outer ring (Wong, 1992). In China, psychiatric care is largely the concern of the family, the state and collectives.

The family

"Certain unique structural features of the Chinese family make it the deep structure of the society and, to a large extent, dictate the practices and behaviours of Chinese society and the Chinese." (Lin Nan, 1988, p. 71)

The family is the first source of help for most Chinese people. Only if the family cannot cope will people turn to others. However, the government does not encourage this, wishing people to be self-sufficient whenever possible to reduce the burden on the state. Families in turn are very often unwilling to seek outside help because it is viewed as demeaning and stigmatising. However, changes in society since 1949 have been mirrored in family structure and could be argued to have affected the family's ability to look after its own. The common notion of the large extended Chinese family living under one roof is increasingly inaccurate. The most common form is the nuclear family. About 60% of rural families are nuclear, as are around 70% of urban families (Lau, 1993). In addition, family size has been shrinking. Between 1982 and 1990 the average household size went from 4.41 to 3.96. Thus, as is the pattern in Western families, there are fewer and fewer people to share the burden of caring for young, old, sick and disabled family members.

Chow (1987) suggests that there is a different consensus among Western and Chinese cultures about why help should be given to the weak and vulnerable and what results should be expected, based partly on their different ideas about the individual's place in the world. For the Chinese, a person is part of a system that starts with the family and through them is connected to wider levels of society. The acceptance of the need to look after those who cannot fend for themselves is not because of a perception of shared humanity, but stems from an extension of the rights and responsibilities that everyone should have as a member of a family. Thus the Chinese have always emphasised the need to look after family members first. Caring for strangers is not a notion that sits very easily in Chinese culture.

The workplace

The primacy of the workplace in the lives of the majority of Chinese people must be stressed. Jobs are not usually chosen; they are allocated or possibly inherited from one or other parent. A very wide range of benefits is provided by the *danwei* either free or at a heavily subsidised rate. These vary from place to place but can include housing, nursery schools, residential accommodation for the elderly, recreational facilities and subsidised food. Without a *danwei*, an individual lacks a 'passport' to the social world. Walder (1986) gives a very full account of the function of the *danwei* system.

The Chinese constitution reflects this emphasis on work. Article 42 states that "citizens of the People's Republic of China have a right as well as a duty to work". Article 6 concludes "the system of socialist public ownership supersedes the system of exploitation of man by man; it applies the principle of 'from each according to his ability, to each according to his work'". This is a quotation from Engels, which is said by him to typify the welfare situation in socialism before the ideal state of communism is achieved.

Mishra (1981, p. 133) claims that "central to the socialist view of welfare is the notion 'to each according to his needs'". He goes on to say (p.137) in relation to the structures in capitalist societies through which welfare needs are met, "in the Soviet Union and in socialist societies generally, neither fiscal benefits nor occupational provision is of comparable scope and significance"[in comparison with the state]. In relation to China this statement is true of fiscal benefits but is grossly inaccurate regarding occupational welfare.

One is forced to examine previously accepted common wisdom. It is supposed to be the exploitative capitalist system that is geared to let the weakest and most vulnerable perish and to define an individual's worth by a capacity for work. If the Chinese truly enforce 'to each according to his work' then those who are handicapped or disabled to an extent that they cannot work are very severely disadvantaged in their capacity to claim the rights of citizenship. We should not be surprised to learn that one of the major emphases in welfare work is the provision of occupation for people with a handicap.

There are two major drawbacks to the provision of welfare benefits via the workplace. First, it discriminates against those who do not have work, who may well be those who need welfare assistance most. In the last ten years, following the introduction of the 'open-door' economic policy, China has had a problem with unemployment and underemployment. Many industries are grossly overstaffed because of the state's responsibility to provide work for all. Once the emphasis turned to profit, enterprises became more cost conscious and tried to avoid carrying surplus employees, which has certainly had a deleterious effect on working opportunities for people with a mental illness in the last ten years.

Second, the 'open-door' policy has led to a division between the more prosperous coastal provinces, rich in resources and connections, like Guangzhou, Fujian and Zhejiang, and the interior provinces, like Gansu and Guangxi, where conditions are very poor and likely to remain so.

The State

In China, the profession of social work is almost unknown. However, many of the typical functions of social work such as the care of the old, young and handicapped who have no one else to care for them must still be performed, with or without trained workers (Pearson & Phillips, 1994*a*).

By the end of 1991, the various welfare institutions of different sorts throughout the country (40 992 in number), provided 828 000 beds (Wong, 1994). The central government's responsibility in this area is borne by the Ministry of Civil Affairs. However, as Wong points out, 95.2 % of all welfare homes are *not* run by the Ministry and the burden of coping with increased demands for care has fallen more and more to the local areas. Despite this, the Ministry of Civil Affairs is relevant in our context because it provides a significant number of psychiatric beds and community-based services (where they exist) for people with a mental illness.

The Ministry of Civil Affairs

The current Ministry of Civil Affairs was established in 1978. In 1991, its total budget was 625 billion yuan, or 1.65% of total national expenditure (*Zhongguo Shehui Bao*, 13 October 1992), a minute amount indicative of the low status its work is given. Civil affairs expenditure as a proportion of the national budget has not exceeded 2% since 1966 (Wong, 1994). The Ministry's prime responsibility is to take care of the 'three have-nots'; that is to say people who are without a home, without support and without a means of livelihood and who are consequently more or less destitute. This would include providing institutional care for the elderly, persons of all ages with a physical or mental handicap, those suffering from a mental illness, children and infants. They are also charged with the care of veterans and the surviving families of revolutionary martyrs.

The decision that the Civil Affairs Department of the Ministry of Home Affairs (as it was then) should provide psychiatric hospitals for the 'three have-nots' (or 'three-nos') patients was taken at the Fourth Conference on Civil Affairs Work in 1958 (*Chinese Civil Affairs Historical Records*, 1986). The impetus for this decision seems to have come from the First National Conference on Mental Health, held the same year in Nanjing (Zhang Dejiang, 1987). Prior to that the Ministry of Home Affairs had provided shelters for destitute people with a mental illness who were found wandering in the streets. These shelters provided food and accommodation but little in the way of treatment. By 1964 there were 203 mental hospitals run by Civil Affairs Departments all over the country. Traditionally, there has been a division of labour between the Ministry of Civil Affairs and the Ministry of Public Health in the provision of psychiatric hospitals. The former takes acute patients who cannot afford to pay for treatment, as well as the majority of long-term patients.

Civil affairs departments at the local level also organise and run productive welfare enterprises. In 1991, they were responsible nationally for 5776 out of a total of 43 758 enterprises employing a total of 701 000 people with a disability. The combined turnover was 41 260 000 renminbi (*Zhongguo Shehui Bao*, 13 October, 1992). These small factories are supposed to provide productive work for those with a handicap who still have some working ability but who would not be able to manage in open employment. In 1988, the then Minister of Civil Affairs declared that "great efforts must be made for the development of factories employing the handicapped", which was entirely consistent with the emphasis placed on the obligation of the state to provide work, and the duty of the citizen to perform productive labour (Cui, 1988, p. 175). However, these welfare factories hardly, if ever, offer employment to people with a mental illness, another instance of the fear they generate, even in people who should know better.

In 1980, the Ministry of Finance and the Ministry of Civil Affairs issued a *Joint Circular On The Payment Of Income Tax by Welfare Production Enterprises Operated By Civil Affairs Departments.* This entitled any factory with disabled workers making up more than 35% of its workforce to be designated a welfare factory and be given certain tax benefits. A further circular was issued in 1984 by the Ministry of Finance concerning *Tax Exemption Matters For Social Welfare Production Enterprises Operated By Civil Affairs Departments.* Under the new policy, eligible units benefited from additional relief from product tax, value added tax and turnover tax (Wong & MacQuarrie, 1986). It is these tax concessions that have been largely responsible for the increase in welfare factories and enterprises over the last ten years. For instance, in Guangzhou there are many welfare factories of different kinds and sizes. Those that make a profit subsidise those that do not. Wong (1993) points out that since 1988 welfare factories have run into grave financial difficulties, with many of them, particularly in the state sector, running at a loss – victims of the changing economic climate and the increasing emphasis on enterprise, self-sufficiency and profit.

Health policy

"The state develops medical and health services, promotes modern medicine and traditional Chinese medicine, encourages and supports the setting up of various medical and health facilities by the rural economic collectives, state enterprises and undertakings and neighbourhood organizations and promotes public health activities of a mass character to promote the people's health. The state develops physical culture and promotes mass sports activities to build up the people's physique" (Article 21, *The Constitution of the People's Republic of China*, 1982).

Ideas about psychiatric care have to fit into a wider framework of health policy generally, an area in which the Chinese government since 1949 has enjoyed considerable success. In 1949, China was known as the sick man of Asia, with a life expectancy of 32 (World Bank, 1984). By 1985 life expectancy was 71 for women and 68 for men (World Bank, 1989). It was clear to the Communist government that improving the nation's health could not be done solely by providing expensive curative health facilities.

In 1950, The Ministry of Public Health called the First National Health Conference which laid down the principles that still guide the provision of health services today. These were that medicine should serve the workers, peasants and soldiers (and not an elite); that preventative health care should take precedence over curative medicine; that Chinese medicine should be integrated with Western scientific medicine; and that health work should be combined with mass movements.

In addition, as a means of encouraging the rational use of scarce resources, a system of 'referring upwards' was developed. Thus, village doctors were supposed to refer difficult cases to the county level hospital, who in turn would send cases beyond their competence to city or provincial level hospitals. This system could always be subverted by those with power and connections (*guanxi*) but worked reasonably well until the 1980s. Once people became richer and health insurance less common and/or less generous, people chose to go the best hospital they could afford, independent of the severity of their complaint.

Achievements following these precepts have been remarkable, to the extent that, for good or ill, China's health profile looks increasingly like those in the more industrialised countries of the West (Hillier, 1988; Henderson, 1990; World Bank, 1992). However, this approach has never really addressed the issues presented by serious mental disorder, with its acute episodes and all too often chronic course. Serious mental disorder remains no more than peripheral to the health policy agenda. There was a gap of 28 years between the first national conference on mental health policy issues in Nanjing in 1958 and the second in Shanghai in 1986.

Prevalence of severe mental disorder and psychiatric facilities

In 1987 a large and comprehensive survey of handicapped people was carried out. The results indicated that 10 million people in China suffered from mental illnesses of various kinds. This surely ought to convince policy makers of the potential of mental illness to have a negative effect on the health of the masses and that dealing with it should be approached with the same energy as was brought to bear on schistosomiasis or malaria.

The most reliable figures concerning the incidence of mental illness in China come from the Twelve Regions Survey carried out in 1982, with the help of the World Health Organization (Coordinating Committee, 1986). This survey found a point prevalence rate for schizophrenia of 6.06 per 1000 in the urban areas and 3.42 per 1000 in the rural areas. However, there is such a variation in the point prevalence rates within the 12 urban and

12 rural areas selected as to throw some doubt on the accuracy of the results (Cheung, 1991). The sample was based on 500 urban and 500 rural households. Given that the incidence of schizophrenia is generally lower in rural areas and that 75% (not 50%, as in the sample) of Chinese people are officially classified as rural dwellers, this may have had an effect on overall prevalence rates. As they stand, these figures are comparable with those in Western countries and Taiwan (Jablensky, 1988). However, the prevalence rates for affective disorder, ranging from 0.37 to 0.89 per thousand, are much lower than found elsewhere. According to the Twelve Region Survey (Coordinating Committee, 1986), schizophrenia is seven times more prevalent in China than affective disorders, while the worldwide rates for schizophrenia and manic-depressive disorder are quite similar (Cheung, 1991). This finding is almost certainly because of a tendency for Chinese psychiatrists to under-diagnose depression and over-diagnose schizophrenia (Yan *et al*, 1984; Cheung, 1991).

The WHO project on schizophrenia (Sartorius *et al*, 1986) demonstrated that the prevalence rates for the disease were lower in underdeveloped and rural areas and that the course of schizophrenia was milder and the prognosis better in developing countries. It could be argued that this profile would fit China, a predominantly rural country. The lower prevalence rate in the rural areas in the Twelve Centre Epidemiological Survey seems to offer some support for this view.

A number of authors have suggested that part of the difference in the course of the illness between the developed and underdeveloped countries may be due to social factors (LeFley, 1986; Jablensky, 1988; Leff, 1988). The two issues most frequently mentioned are, first, larger families, which are presumed to be more accepting and less critical because the burden of caring for someone with schizophrenia can be spread more thinly. Second, the greater availability of ordinary and socially meaningful work (agriculture) within the capacity of someone with a vulnerability to psychosis. Unfortunately, there seems to be no reliable information on the course of schizophrenia in China, so it is not possible to know whether the general findings of the WHO research apply. One finding from the Twelve Centre Epidemiological Survey does suggest that large family size offers some protection against the more severe manifestations of schizophrenia; prevalence was lowest among large families and highest in nuclear and medium-sized ones (Coordinating Committee, 1986).

It is very difficult to obtain reliable figures concerning the provision of psychiatric facilities. This is partly because of the logistical problems of compiling reliable information in such a large and developmentally diverse country. It is also to do with the air of secrecy which surrounds much official information in China. This is compounded by the fact that mental illness is such a stigmatising condition – not only for the individual but also the national character – that there is a reluctance to publish statistics because it is thought that revealing such information puts the country in a bad light.

Three ministries are largely responsible for providing psychiatric hospitals and formulating policy on psychiatric care. These are the Ministry of Public Health, the Ministry of Civil Affairs and the Ministry of Public Security (the police). The precise division of responsibility may vary between them from place to place. However, as a general rule the Ministry of Public Health runs hospitals that deal largely with those who are acutely ill. The Ministry of Civil Affairs takes in patients who cannot afford the fees charged by the Ministry of Public Health and is also responsible for more of the chronic care hospitals. The Ministry of Public Security runs the forensic psychiatric hospitals (Pearson, 1992*b*).

The *1992 Statistical Year Book of China* claims that there are 449 psychiatric hospitals in China, providing 89 000 beds, but it seems likely that this only takes into account the facilities run by the Ministry of Public Health. An internal document on rehabilitation reports that the Ministry of Civil Affairs is responsible for 35 000 beds which constitutes over 33% of all hospital beds for those with a mental illness, and that 85% of their beds are occupied by patients with a chronic mental illness.

A pamphlet produced by the West China University of Medical Sciences in 1990 states that there are 473 psychiatric institutions under the Ministry of Public Health, 190 under the Ministry of Civil Affairs, 81 under the Ministry of Industry and Mining, 23 under the Ministry of Public Security, 24 under the armed forces and 12 under local collectives. Unfortunately, this pamphlet does not distinguish between hospitals, research institutes, departments of psychiatry in medical schools, psychiatric wards in general hospitals and freestanding clinics. Nor have they obtained information about the number of beds involved. Furthermore, none of these sets of figures take into account the relatively recent phenomenon of private 'hospitals' for those with a mental illness. The 1987 document *Opinions About Strengthening Mental Health Work* (discussed in more detail below) reported that there were then six beds per 1000 patients. It seems likely that nobody knows exactly how many psychiatric hospital beds there are and what kinds of patients are occupying them. A best 'guesstimate' for the number of beds may be between 100 000 and 120 000.

Policy at provincial and local level is still implemented through the mechanism of the 'three man leading groups' mentioned in Chapter 1. These groups are supposed to provide coordination at the different levels and a degree of professional guidance and supervision of lower levels by higher levels. In some areas, like Shanghai, it has been very successful (Zhang *et al,* 1994). In others the system is moribund. Even where this system works well, it is still largely a mechanism for enforcing 'top-down' policy decisions rather than formulating policy and developing services at a local level. Like many other systems in China, much depends on the enthusiasm and quality of the people involved. Because central government funding is so limited, Beijing has little leverage in ensuring that the provinces carry out national policy. The issue of financing takes on an increasingly important role in the decision about who gets what and where.

Mental health care funding

It is a common, but erroneous, impression that because China has a socialist/communist political system it upholds universalist principles of accessibility and provides services free to all its citizens. This is not the case. From the very beginning of the People's Republic there was never any question that medical services would be provided free to all citizens. Resources then and now do not permit it. The official view is that the state's responsibility is to provide basic preventive services while curative health services should be paid for by the consumer. Over the last decade, the move from a centralised economy to a socialist market economy (which bears many resemblances to capitalism) has emphasised this demarcation. Hospitals are increasingly having to rely on their own income-generating abilities, rather than grants from the government. Grants, for instance, cover basic staff salaries but not the bonuses which make up between 30 to 50% of take-home pay.

This has increased the pressure to admit patients and keep them as long as possible, especially if they are a reliable source of income. Phillips (1990) has demonstrated that length of stay for patients in his sample of psychiatric hospitals was related to whether the patient had health insurance rather than the type or severity of their illness. Individual treatments (recreational, music, and laser therapies, for instance) are often charged separately at a large cumulative cost to the patient. As will be discussed in Chapter 4, this inevitably affects the provision and financing of community-based services, which do not generate income on anything like the same scale and yet often rely on hospital-based doctors for supervision and support. In some hospitals, individual doctors are given a target monthly income that they must generate. If they fail to meet their target all the staff on that ward are financially penalised. Thus peer pressure is brought to bear in order to maintain personal and hospital income.

Admission to a psychiatric ward in 1994 costs on average between 700 and 1000 yuan a month (but may be as high as 2000 yuan) and a month's deposit is expected in advance. This is approximately the same as the annual income for a rural household. If a patient is not covered by health insurance (see below), costs can be crippling. Much needed care may simply be unaffordable. Gu *et al* (1993) in their study of health care utilisation in rural areas found that the level of charges deterred people from seeking hospital care, even when it was recommended by a doctor. The problem was particularly noticeable among the poorest of the rural population and in the remoter villages. The thrust of Mao Zedong's health policy, particularly during the Cultural Revolution, was to bring more and better health care to the rural areas. Even with all his authority, and the use of draconian measures, it was never easy to do. Now, since the beginning of the reform period, state spending on the rural medical service, as a percentage of the nation's medical budget, has fallen from 21% in 1978 to 10% in 1991 (*China Daily*, 3 May 1994). In October 1994 the Minister of Health, in his national health report to the National People's Congress Standing Committee, pledged that 75 million renminbi would be allocated by the central government over the next six years, mainly to be spent on establishing medical centres in remote, poverty-stricken areas (*Beijing Review*, 7 November 1994)

Health insurance

Health insurance is the way through which citizens are helped to meet medical costs but there are very significant differences between the urban and rural schemes. The Labour Insurance Regulations for urban workers were first promulgated in 1951, and their basic structure remains the same. The regulations cover all workers and staff employed in state operated enterprises, mines and railways. The entire scheme is a noncontributory one and the enterprises are responsible for shouldering the whole burden of sickness and disablement benefit, maternity leave and pensions (Chow, 1988). Increasingly, many are finding this difficult to do.

The rules, which are still in operation in many places, entitled workers injured at work to medical treatment at designated hospitals and clinics; wages in full throughout the period of treatment; and 60–100 % of wages as a pension when certified to be wholly disabled. Injury, sickness and disablement not sustained at work are also provided for, with 60–100% of wages being payable for up to six months and in some places longer. Dependent family members of the worker would also be eligible for sickness benefits. There is also a government insurance that covers government employees (Pearson, 1995).

As can be seen, these provisions are generous. However, these regulations discriminate against urban workers who are not employed by large enterprises, as the regulations apply only to enterprises employing 100 or more. An additional problem of recent genesis is that of individual workers in the urban areas who have no labour insurance protection. One source puts the number at 20 million (Wei Xingwu, 1988). In addition, there is the problem of the 'floating' population of migrants, usually from rural areas, who leave their place of registration and go to the cities to seek work. According to Siu & Li (1993), such people account for six per cent of the total population. They, of course, have no social security protection. Many enterprises are attempting to cut back on their health insurance obligations. Some will offer workers an interest free loan, others offer to pay only a proportion of hospital costs and so on.

Initially, the enterprises paid their benefit contributions into a labour insurance fund which provided some element of risk sharing. However, the labour insurance scheme administered by the All China Federation of Trade Unions ceased to operate during the chaos of the Cultural Revolution. In 1969 the Ministry of Finance issued an order that the relevant benefits would be paid directly by the enterprises as labour insurance expenses. This in effect discontinued the labour insurance funds and led to benefits being paid directly out of operating expenses, thus destroying the re-distributive and risk sharing element. At the time this caused little concern, because there were few retired workers.

In retrospect, the results of this policy have been detrimental. Very few enterprises created their own benefits fund. Consequently, the longer established the enterprise, the greater the number of retired, disabled or sick workers whose benefits have to come out of the operating expenses. This puts the newly established enterprises in an advantageous position because with fewer retired, disabled or chronically sick workers they have more money to re-invest in equipment, research and so on (Wei Xingwu, 1988). Chow (1994) discusses developments in the Labour Insurance Regulations since the mid-1980s and the introduction of contributory schemes with regard to unemployment insurance and old age pensions, a radical change from the previous policy that such benefits would be the responsibility of employers, not employees. However, such developments have not been widely applied to health insurance (Chow, 1994).

Cooperative health insurance

Chow (1988) estimates that the benefits of the labour insurance programme are unavailable to at least 80% of workers and their families in China. What arrangements then are made for the peasants who form the majority of the population?

The answer is supposed to be what is known as cooperative health insurance. The idea was first proposed by the Nationalist government in their first Three Year Plan (1931–1934), although there is no evidence that they acted on it (Lucas, 1982). The Communist government first mooted this scheme in 1958 but pursued the idea seriously only in 1968. It was based on the notion that there should be risk sharing at the commune level (now known as townships). Communes usually consisted of 20 000–50 000 people. Under this system, each commune or brigade member paid a standard fee which then went into a collective pool out of which medicines, a portion of hospital costs, equipment and 'barefoot doctors' remuneration were paid.

This system was considerably less generous than the health insurance provided for urban workers. It also had inherent problems in that it did not contribute to the redistribution of resources from the richer to poorer areas. Healthier peasants in the communes were reluctant to subsidise those who were heavier users of the scheme. The success of cooperative health insurance had always depended on generating an annual surplus. Thus financing was now forever uncertain and some of the schemes were unable to meet their obligations.

Personal observation, confirmed by a number of authors (Chen & Tuan, 1983; Hillier & Jewell, 1983; Chow, 1988; Henderson, 1990), suggests that the system of cooperative health insurance has been severely undermined by the dismantling of the commune system since the decision taken at the Third Plenum of the Communist Party in 1979 to let peasants cultivate their own plots in line with the 'open door' policy. Without the communally organised finances at brigade (village) or commune (township) level there is no basis for cooperative insurance because, on the whole, families prefer to bear the risk themselves.

In 1975 an estimated 84.5% of the rural Chinese population was covered by collective financing of health care. By 1985, this had fallen to 39.9% (Zhu *et al*, 1989) and by 1989 only 5% of the rural population were covered (Gu *et al*, 1992). Zhu *et al* (1989) point out that the decline cannot all be attributed to the effects of the 'contract responsibility system', because the changes in rural areas have not been uniform. Local community leaders in their study felt that the government had stopped actively promoting communal health insurance and village doctors (as barefoot doctors are now known), and that this was contributing substantially towards the system's decline. Outside the larger enterprises, the system of cooperative health insurance is in disarray and many families in China are left to carry the burden of hospital charges unassisted (*China Daily*, 3 May 1994). The government recognises that there is a problem and in 1988 the Ministry of Public Health constituted an Expert Commission on Health Policy and Management to assess the situation and develop viable policy options (Gu *et al*, 1993).

A measure of the severity of the problem is that the Chinese government is seriously considering opening the Chinese market to American insurance firms and is turning to them for advice. A seminar was held in Beijing in May 1994 hosted by the People's Insurance Company of China to which 16 leading US insurance companies were invited (*China Daily*, 26 May 1994). It is difficult to see how such a strategy will assist those most seriously in need. This is particularly so in the case of those suffering from chronic disorders, like severe mental illness, that insurance companies are notoriously reluctant to cover.

Medical private practice

Private practice was strongly discouraged from 1949 onwards, although at times it was the only way that a number of people, particularly in the rural areas, could gain access to any curative health care at all. In 1949 there were 6669 private practitioners; 2829 in 1956; 1514 in 1965; 506 in 1981; 432 in 1984 (*China News Analysis*, 1985, No. 1296). Since the contract responsibility system was introduced, private practice has gradually re-emerged. In 1980 the State Council approved a report of the Ministry of Public Health allowing doctors to practise privately (*People's Daily*, 6

September 1985, p. 4). This seems to have had little effect until 1985 when 80 200 were registered (9200 in the cities and 71 000 in the countryside, 78% of whom were practitioners of Chinese traditional medicine (*China News Analysis*, 1985, No. 296; Hillier, 1988).

On April 25, 1985, the State Council approved a *Report of the Ministry of Public Health on Some Policy Questions Concerning the Reform of Health Work*. Among other reforms, this permits individual health practitioners to open hospitals and clinics and practice medicine independently. The practice has extended to the psychiatric sector. Doctors at Anding Hospital told me that there were at least two small private psychiatric hospitals in the suburbs where the major qualifications of the staff were said to be well-developed muscles. An article in the *China Daily* (18 March 1989) reported that there were 18 privately run psychiatric hospitals in Beijing providing 2000 beds. According to figures given in the same article this would constitute 40% of all available psychiatric beds in Beijing. Apart from concerns about standards of care, a burgeoning private sector will almost certainly drain doctors from the state sector to the more lucrative private sector.

Where do the poor go?

In a speech given at the Second National Mental Health Conference, the Vice Minister of Civil Affairs, Zhang Dejiang (1987) argued that:

"We must face reality and develop self-pay care. With the increase in living standards of the people and the continuous development of society there are fewer and fewer mental patients who have no family to go to, no financial resources and no supportive network. There are more and more who are doing nothing productive for society but who do have family support. To work with this reality and to cope with the need of society and expectation of the people we broke the old way of working and shattered the original idea of the 'three have-nots'. This eliminates problems for society, the patients' families and the *danweis* and has got very good results. According to initial statistics, at present over 50 % of mental patients cared for by the Civil Affairs Ministry are self-funded. Experience illustrates that the advent of self-pay care has been deeply welcomed by families and *danweis* and has made the hospitals full of life and activity."

This is all very well for those who can pay; but it has changed the basis of hospitalisation – bearing in mind that a psychiatric bed is a relatively scarce resource – from those who need it most to those who can afford it. It discriminates in favour of those who are covered by the Labour Insurance Regulations and against those who are peasants. It also does not address the question of what happens to those people who need long-term care. The 'three have-nots' are the totally destitute. But there are hundreds of millions of people in China who, for various reasons, have not been able to benefit from the economic reforms and who are just plain poor. They have families, means of support and a livelihood but that does not put them in a position to pay very high hospital fees. Some hospitals in the Ministry of Civil Affairs network operate a system of fee remission for the poorer self-pay patients but many do not. The introduction of a fee income system means better bonuses for staff and perhaps a more pleasant type of patient to treat. It may even lead to the upgrading of hospitals, which will, of course, benefit patients. But it is done at the expense of poor and chronically ill patients.

Medical personnel

With the exception of some of the more famous hospitals in the major cities, psychiatric hospitals in China are staffed almost exclusively by doctors and nurses. Occupational therapists, social workers and psychologists are virtually nonexistent (Pearson & Phillips, 1994a). Study and training opportunities for the latter two groups ceased in the mid-1950s when the teaching of social sciences in the universities was banned for political reasons. The lack of a social science perspective in psychiatric treatment and care has had a deleterious effect, not only in terms of the relentlessly biological model of care espoused by most doctors, but also in the understanding of ward dynamics and the iatrogenic effects of institutional life. Psychologists, where they exist, are mostly employed to carry out psychological tests (an important potential source of ward income) and are not involved in treatment.

The government has shown some interest in developing social work programmes. For instance, in 1988 the Sociology Department at Beijing University was given one million yuan to develop some social work courses (*China Daily*, 12 December 1988). However, such efforts have had only limited effects. They are not focused on people who work with those suffering from a mental illness, and students allocated to quasi-social work positions after graduation appear to suffer a crisis of identification and confusion about their role (Pearson & Phillips, 1994a).

Doctors

The 1931 *League of Nations Health Organization Report on Medical Schools in China* recommended a two level system of medical education for China: national medical colleges at university level to produce 'high grade physicians' and experimentally upgraded provincial level medical schools to train a larger number of medical practitioners (Lucas, 1982).

This two-level system of education is still in place in China (World Bank, 1992). From its instigation, it has been the subject of a 'quality versus quantity' debate. It was argued that with limited resources and a vast population, China could not afford to train all the necessary medical staff to the highest level. It was therefore better to have larger numbers, adequately trained to deal with common illnesses and who could recognise what was beyond their capacity, so that the patient could be referred if necessary to more sophisticated facilities. Medical training at both levels includes very little on psychiatry, probably no more than two to four weeks, with little or no exposure to patients.

The issue of equity and the rural–urban divide was of particular importance to the Communist government. Mao Zedong formed the opinion that the Ministry of Health was not doing enough to provide doctors and services to the rural areas. Furthermore, they also represented an elitist bastion of medical power, favouring lengthy training, research and high technology. He issued his famous directive of June 26, 1965, which became the foundation of all policy initiatives in the health sector for the next ten years. It is worth quoting at some length:

"Tell the Ministry of Public Health that it only works for 15% of the total population of the country and that this 15% is mainly composed of lords, while the broad masses of the peasants do not get any medical treatment. First they don't have any doctors. Second they don't have any medicine. The Ministry of Public Health is not a Ministry of Public Health for the People, so why not change its name to the Ministry of Urban Health, the Ministry of Lord's Health, or even to the Ministry of Urban Lord's Health?...Medical education should be reformed. There's no need to read so many books. In medical education there is no need to accept only higher middle school graduates, It will be enough to give three years to graduates from higher primary schools. They would then study and raise their standards mainly through practice. If this kind of doctor is sent down to the countryside, even if they don't have much talent, they would be better than quacks and witchdoctors and the villages would be better able to afford to keep them. The more books one reads the more stupid one gets...We should leave behind in the city a few of the less able doctors who graduated one or two years ago and the others should all go to the countryside...In medical and health work put the emphasis on the countryside." (Quoted in Lampton, 1977, pp. 185–186)

Chen & Tuan (1983) discuss the question of people entering the health care system with no training at all. They say that there were essentially two reasons for this. First, that during the Cultural Revolution many people with no training were given jobs because of nepotism and factionalism. Secondly, since 1978, with increasing unemployment, county and municipal governments have resorted to the practice of letting children 'inherit' their parents' jobs. Chen & Tuan claim that since 1966, 42% of persons recruited into the nation's health care system had no prior training in health care whatsoever. In Jilin province, in 1980, 4007 out of a total of 6009 persons recruited into the provincial health care system had no prior training.

In June 1981 the Chinese Communist Party Organisational Department and the Party Committee of the Ministry of Health issued a joint statement calling on CCP committees at all levels to "strive not to or to appoint as few as possible" persons without proper training to the health care system. They were told that in filling vacancies, graduates of the medical colleges or the middle level medical schools should be looked upon as the major source of candidates. Chen & Tuan (1983) emphasise that the position has improved somewhat since this circular was issued. For a variety of reasons, including being classified during the Cultural Revolution as the 'stinking number nine class', doctors do not enjoy the independence of action and respect that their counterparts in the West take for granted.

Specialist training

As far as can be ascertained, there is not now and never has been any national system of accredited postgraduate specialist training in psychiatry in China (Liu & Jia, 1994). There are doctors who specialise in psychiatry and who, at least in Beijing, study for a Master's Degree in medicine. Postgraduate training is reported to have been initiated in psychiatric hospitals in Shanghai, Changsha, Siping, Chengdu, Beijing and Nanjing (Xia & Zhang, 1981). It will be many years before this limited amount of training can be expected to have an effect. The more usual system of training seems to be based on learning by observation, through apprenticeship to older experts who in turn have learned what they know through many years of practice.

It has to be remembered that in China newly qualified doctors are not free to choose the area in which they specialise. The decision is taken by the personnel office at the training institution. At one time, in the late 1970s and early 1980s, the system was very inflexible and students had no choice at all. Gradually, the system has become more flexible. For instance, students who pay their own fees, about 20%, are free to choose their own job. Currently, state aided students are allowed to express their preferences about where to work. The higher their marks in the final exams, the more likely they are to get their first or second choice.

Geography also enters the equation and students may trade off speciality against location. On the whole, they prefer to work in large cities, so a student might well accept a job in psychiatry in Beijing rather than a position in surgery in Gansu. A migration of the most skilled health personnel to urban centres and higher-level institutions has been predicted in a recent report on health in China (World Bank, 1992). This is seen as the consequence of policies, likely to be implemented in the 1990s, of a greater liberalisation in the job market and greater autonomy in setting wage levels.

Psychiatry is a very unpopular area to work in and at least the current system of allocating jobs has protected it from being grossly understaffed, even if the doctors are reluctant recruits with poor professional morale. The Ministry of Public Health has for some years been considering the advisability of permitting free choice, but as yet has not implemented the change in policy. If this ever happens, it is almost certain to precipitate a crisis in staffing psychiatric hospitals.

There are nationally accepted hierarchical grades for doctors and provincially organised exams must be passed before a doctor is eligible to proceed to the next grade. All exams have two components, one generic and the other in the doctor's speciality. In the late 1980s rules were promulgated to try and ensure that standards were even and procedures uniform from province to province.

A newly qualified doctor must spend seven years at the first level before being permitted to take the examination to qualify for consideration for promotion to the second level. The exam to reach the third level requires another five years of practise to become eligible. Doctors are not allowed to enter themselves for the examinations and must be sponsored and nominated by their hospital. This obviously leaves room for favouritism and influence.

The Ministry of Public Health and the Ministry of Civil Affairs set their own exams, which are supposed to be equivalent to each other. The status of each grade is the same in each ministry, although salaries may be generally higher in the Ministry of Public Health.

Passing the exam does not bring automatic promotion. Younger doctors often have to wait for older doctors to retire or to be promoted in their turn before a vacancy at their appropriate level of qualification becomes available. Thus expertise in any speciality tends to be acquired through self-study if the person is enthusiastic and motivated, or is assumed to exist if the doctor has worked in that area a long time. If a Chinese doctor begins a sentence "In my thirty years of experience" it is expected to preclude further argument. And it usually does.

Village doctors

In addition to the two kinds of doctor already described, there is a third type, currently known as a village doctor. As the name suggests, they staff the clinics in the villages, looking after basic health care, immunisation programmes, and supposedly providing a referral link upwards in the medical system for illnesses they are not capable of handling. They have their genesis in the 'barefoot' doctors of the Maoist era.

Mao's health strategy contained three elements including 'walking on two legs', which meant giving equal emphasis to the 'treasure-house' of Chinese medicine and not relying so much on Western medicine; changing the focus of practice to the rural areas; and training doctors who had just three years of primary schooling. Barefoot doctors were first mentioned in 1955, in a commune in Henan implementing a cooperative medical system (Zhu *et al*, 1989). The medical schools closed down in 1966; many of the staff were criticised, beaten, imprisoned and the majority were sent down to the rural areas. In the same year an official report first mentioned barefoot doctors:

> "A new type of peasant physician who is both a medical worker and a peasant is coming into being in every part of China. With a current campaign to extend the medical services... group after group of city doctors have been going into the countryside and large numbers of graduates of city medical colleges have been assigned to work in county hospitals or commune clinics. But this is only part of the answer and in order to ensure that adequate medical and health services become available to peasants everywhere part-study part-secondary medical schools

are being set up to train secondary medical personnel amongst the peasants locally." (quoted in Hillier & Jewell, 1983, p. 362)

Barefoot doctors had variable amounts of training that ranged from 6 weeks to 18 months (spread over a period of years). They were expected to be, at the least, responsible for sanitation and hygiene work, vaccination and inoculation, maternal and child health and treating common and minor illnesses. Much of their training was based at county level hospitals, which usually had an intermediate-level trained doctor on the staff. Barefoot doctors were selected and financed by their production brigades and were expected to continue to work part-time in the fields. The original idea was that they were a link in the referral chain; but by about 1970 the press were lauding the feats of barefoot doctors who performed advanced surgery and treated difficult cases, and this has to be interpreted as a sign of official policy. Between 1966 and 1976 over two million people were trained as barefoot doctors (Chen & Tuan, 1983).

However, by the early- and mid-1970s when people were more free to speak out, deep concern was expressed about the adequacy of the service provided by barefoot doctors. In 1973 Deng Xiaoping suggested that barefoot doctors should "go from barefoot to sandals and from cloth shoes to leather shoes" (Hillier & Jewell, 1983). The Sidels report that Deng once walked out of a showing of a propaganda film on the work of barefoot doctors which he thought to be portraying them going well beyond their levels of competence (Sidel & Sidel, 1982) The expectations of many of the people about the quality of care to which they are entitled have since been raised, and many are in a position to distinguish between good and bad value. Among other things, it was the dissatisfaction of the ordinary people with the quality of the barefoot doctors that led to their upgrading in training, status and salary.

The National People's Congress held in 1980 passed a resolution changing the name of the barefoot doctors to the equivalent of the American term 'paramedic'. Since about 1978 the numbers of barefoot doctors have dropped significantly, partly due to problems in funding, lack of status and insufficient salary. Standards of training have been raised. By 1986, 40% of barefoot doctors had attained the level of medical school graduates, and upon passing a qualifying examination were certified as village or country doctors (Huang, 1988; Zhu *et al*, 1989). The majority of village doctors now charge fees and earn a proportion of their income by selling drugs. Many village clinics have become private (Gu *et al*, 1993).

Nurses

Perhaps the most unusual thing about the situation of nurses in China is that there are fewer of them than doctors. According to a report in the *China Daily Business Weekly* (March 8–14, 1992) based on figures from the State Statistical Bureau, by the end of 1991 there were 3.99 million medical doctors and only 1.01 million nurses. The World Bank report on health care in China (1992, p. 98) has this to say:

> "China is currently employing a particularly inefficient approach to nursing care, in effect delegating it 'upward' to physicians rather than developing a skilled professional nursing corps. Most nursing today is provided by secondary school graduates...who have only limited clinical and medical skills. Their functions in hospitals are too often confined to semi-skilled and housekeeping functions."

The report recommends a more nearly equal doctor to nurse ratio and significant quantitative and qualitative improvements in nursing standards.

Bueber (1993*b*) describes psychiatric nursing as a fledgling discipline. The first national psychiatric nursing association was formed in 1990 and is attempting to hold national meetings annually. As yet, there is no journal of psychiatric nursing. Nurses are trained in two or three year programmes in the lower level medical schools, following a basic training that does not include any psychiatry. Older nurses working on a ward may have little or no formal training because of the disruptions caused by the Cultural Revolution, although they may be classified, after a time, as qualified. It is also common to find a high proportion of nurses on wards who would more properly be called 'nurses' aides' in the West. Kincheloe, writing in 1985, states that she was told nurses' training consisted of a two year apprenticeship in a hospital. In locations where there are insufficient nursing personnel, it is possible to become a nurse after working as a nursing aide for five years and then passing an examination (Bueber, 1992). In areas where doctors are scarce, qualified nurses may take examinations to become doctors (Henderson & Cohen, 1984; Bueber, 1992). There are four levels of qualified nurse: registered nurse, advanced nurse, vice-chief nurse and chief nurse (Bueber, 1992). Progression through the hierarchy is dependent on years of experience and passing an examination to qualify for the next level.

Thus a nurse allocated to a psychiatric hospital is unlikely to have either theoretical or practical experience in the area of psychiatric nursing. Because of the stigma and fear associated with this client group, she is also likely to be a very reluctant recruit and bring to her work all the negative, stereotypical beliefs about people with a mental illness common among lay people (Bueber, 1993a; Tousley, 1985). I was told by a senior doctor in Anding Hospital in Beijing that when newly qualified nurses are informed that they have been allocated to psychiatric nursing at the hospital, they are liable to burst into tears and beg to be sent elsewhere.

Bueber (1993a), based on several years experience of being co-head nurse in a Chinese psychiatric hospital, argues that the primary function of psychiatric nurses in China is to guard and control patients, rather than to provide care. As nurses receive no training in psychotherapeutic techniques, building therapeutic relationships with patients is not recognised as an important nursing role. There are no national standards specific for nursing care so the evaluation of psychiatric nurses' performance is based on their ability to make beds, insert urinary catheters and administer intravenous and intramuscular medication.

The low quality of psychiatric nursing in China is a serious impediment to the improvement of psychiatric care both on and off the ward. As in other countries, psychiatric nurses have more face-to-face contact with patients than any one else, and are thus in a position to affect the treatment experience. As yet, the government does not seem to have identified this as a priority area of concern.

The State Council Document of 1987

The Second National Meeting on mental health was held in Shanghai in 1986, jointly called by the three Ministries most concerned with mental health work: Civil Affairs, Public Health and Public Security. This meeting produced the first major assessment of the state of psychiatric care, and guidelines for future directions, in 28 years. The resulting document was approved by the State Council and issued in 1987. It was entitled *Opinions About Strengthening Mental Health Work* and was circulated to all departmental officers concerned in local people's governments in all provinces, autonomous regions and municipalities, with copies to Public Health, Public Security and Civil Affairs Departments in all provinces, autonomous regions, and municipalities. It was accompanied by the message "Please carry it out thoroughly, according to the local situation". As this document has not been made available outside China and has received only little attention in Western sources (Pearson & Phillips, 1994*b*), its contents are presented below in some detail.

The first paragraph is about the achievements in mental health work since the First National Meeting in 1958 in Nanjing, but after that the document is exclusively concerned with problems and what to do about them. The problems are listed as follows:

1. There is insufficient understanding about the importance and urgency of mental health work and "many comrades do not appreciate the internal relationship between mental health work and the construction of socialist spiritual civilization". Insufficient emphasis is put on this work and it lacks support.

2. There is an obvious increase in the occurrence of mental illness. Currently there are more than ten million mental patients in China. With industrialisation and modernisation psychosocial factors associated with mental illness develop continuously. The occurrence rate has increased from 0.7% in the 1970s to 1.54% in the 1980s and is growing. Nearly half of all psychiatric patients experience relapse and cause 'serious danger' to society.

3. There is a serious shortfall in agencies doing mental health work, in hospital beds, funding and manpower. Mental hospital buildings are old, run-down and unsuitable and facilities are primitive. Many of them are built in remote areas far away from the city that they serve. This causes difficulties for patients and relatives and makes management of the hospitals awkward.

(a) The government allocates only half the funds to psychiatric hospitals that they give to general hospitals at the same grade. This means that necessary repairs and upgrading of old equipment cannot be carried out. Because of lack of financial support, community treatment and prevention which has been shown to be very effective cannot be implemented. The most pressing case is that of mental hospitals run by the Ministry of Public Security for those patients who have broken the law and urgently need treatment and confinement. More hospitals cannot be built because of lack of funds and as a consequence these kinds of patients continue to seriously endanger social order.

(b) There are insufficient hospital beds. At present there are only six beds for every 1000 psychiatric patients. As many as 80% of patients are not able to receive treatment and 95% of patients cannot be admitted to hospital. Some patients are chained up at home for years and treated inhumanely. Some enterprises deploy production workers to watch mental patients 24 hours a day in three shifts. Care for psychiatric patients has become a long-term burden for society, enterprises and families.

(c) There is a serious lack of organisation, training and a supply of experienced mental health workers. There are only 6 psychiatrists for every 10 000 mental patients. The ratio between hospital beds and staff is only 1:0.6. The quality of work is poor. Mental health workers are not valued by society and are called doctors for 'loonies'. The heavy workload, high risk, low pay, and unfair assessment of professional requirements and poor promotion prospects make new staff reluctant to join and unsettles the existing staff.

4. The lack of treatment facilities for mental patients means that many of them are living in the community with no treatment or supervision. The trouble and danger caused are quite serious. According to a survey carried out in Jiangsu province, there have been more than 1800 crimes committed by psychiatric patients since 1985. Of these, 130 were murders; 189 people sustaining serious injury; 209 cases of arson; 800 cases of robbery or theft. In many serious crimes mental patients occupy a considerable percentage of the offenders. A female patient from Heilongjiang province crept into the memorial hall to Chairman Mao in Beijing, trying to break the glass coffin. In the oil refinery at Daqing a psychiatric patient caused 100 million yuan's worth of damage by deliberately starting a fire. In Shanghai a patient knocked down and killed 15 pedestrians when driving a car. Other cases involve psychiatric patients displaying their nude bodies, causing shame and trouble, and damaging electricity supplies so that factories and mines have to stop work and production. These are common cases and these frightening facts are enough to illustrate that if we do not have active means to strengthen mental health work then even more serious social problems will occur.

The document continues by pointing out that China is in a new phase of economic development and that improving the mental health of the nation is very important and is "related to social peace, the safety of property and the lives of citizens". Mental health work needs to be put on an 'important agenda' and the following suggestions are made:

1. A joint committee led by the Ministries of Public Health, Public Security and Civil Affairs should be set up to coordinate and guide national mental health work. Personnel from other ministries should also be involved.

2. Mental health work should be incorporated into the construction of a socialist spiritual civilisation and be included in all local plans for development. This would give it the recognition it deserves and the necessary support when the national budget permits.

3. More effort should be put into training to solve the manpower problems. High level medical colleges should add courses on mental health to their programmes. Training in prevention and treatment of psychiatric illness should also be encouraged. Efforts should be made to solve the problem of fair job evaluation and rewards for mental health professionals. Emphasis should be given to strengthening scientific research in mental health.

4. Mental health legislation and forensic psychiatric assessment and treatment facilities should be developed as quickly as possible. A forensic psychiatric assessment committee should be formed as soon as possible by the public security, health and judicial authorities.

5. More facilities should be established for the treatment and community management of people with a mental illness; welfare factories and work stations should be exempted from tax; mental health facilities should be developed by exploring the possibilities for multi-channelled fund raising; generally, community prevention, treatment and management work should be improved; and every effort made to accommodate, treat and manage mental patients.

6. Publicity about the importance of mental health work and to spread scientific knowledge about mental health and illness should be strengthened; everyone should be asked to show recognition of and concern for mental health work, so that all Chinese people can have a good working and living environment, and social, familial and psychological factors which lead to mental illness can be reduced; conditions which help to rehabilitate people with a mental illness back to their own environments should be created.

This is probably the most honest official statement available about the condition of psychiatric services. Clearly, the problems that are faced are similar to those experienced elsewhere: a lack of funds; discrimination against psychiatric hospitals in favour of general hospitals; poor training and an unwillingness to join mental health work; poor terms of service; concern about the potential of some psychiatric patients to seriously disrupt society; lack of understanding and stigmatisation of those with a mental illness from the general public and government officials; a recognition that community services are important, yet a continuing policy emphasis on increasing beds. However, no other country faces the sheer enormity of coordinating and providing services for 1.2 billion people, or as the document says, ten million psychiatric patients.

Yet if this document is supposed to serve as guidance, it can only be described as grossly inadequate. The recommendations constitute little more than a 'wish list', with very little in the way of pragmatic suggestions or operational plans to outline the necessary steps to be taken, people to be influenced and concrete goals to be achieved. Most important, there are no detailed considerations for resource implications, of what the multi-channelled sources of fund raising might consist, or how the burden of finance could be shared between national, provincial and local sources of funding. Other than saying that 'whatever it is, we need more', there are no guidelines as to what number of beds, out-patient facilities and so on there should be per head of population.

Furthermore, one is also left with the impression that the people involved in writing this document were all urban-based. There was no attempt at all to address one of the most serious problems in health service delivery; how to reach the 75% of the population living in rural areas. Nor is there any discussion of how to regulate the supply of drugs in a rational way based on predictions of use, so that the smaller and less well known hospitals are not subject to interrupted supplies.

When a professor of psychiatry, based in Beijing, was asked who decided mental health policy in China, he told me that it was largely up to the Minister of Public Health, who is advised by 16 senior psychiatrists in seven subject areas: child, community, psychosocial aspects, geriatric, forensic, epilepsy and education. Lin (1985) confirms that there is no office or officer in the Ministry of Public Health responsible for mental health. The Beijing professor did not consider that psychiatry receives much priority – an understatement.

Deng Pufang and the disability initiative

The greatest cause for hope in this moribund situation comes from the impetus generated by Deng Pufang in his search for a better deal for China's vast number of people with a handicap. Deng Pufang is the older son of China's Paramount Leader, Deng Xiaoping. During the Cultural Revolution (1966–1976), when his father was branded as a 'capitalist roader', Deng Pufang was thrown out of a third floor window by Red Guards. His back was broken and he has since been confined to a wheelchair.

In 1984 he established the China Welfare Fund for the Disabled and then the China Federation for Disabled People in 1988. He was the prime mover behind the national survey of people with a disability in 1987, the first time China had ever attempted this sort of assessment. Another sign of his success was the promulgation in 1990 of the first *Law of the People's Republic of China on the Protection of Disabled Persons* which was to be implemented from May 1991.

Senior psychiatrists with an interest in rehabilitation realised that climbing on this particular bandwagon was probably their best chance of improving the lot of those with a mental illness. A number of them approached Deng Pufang and he agreed that people with a mental illness could be included as one of the groups of people suffering a disability (Tian *et al*, 1994). Thus, they were included in the 1991 legislation (article 2). Official recognition of that kind is vital in China.

In addition, the 'Deng Pufang connection' led to the formation in 1990 of the Chinese Rehabilitation and Research Association for the Mentally Disabled. It is subsumed under the Chinese Rehabilitation and Research Association for the Disabled, which in turn is part of the China Federation for the Disabled. The 1991 law (article 8) officially recognises the China Federation for the Disabled. It is required to "represent the interests of disabled persons, protect their lawful rights and interests, educate disabled persons and provide service for disabled persons". For the first time, there is a channel through which those interested in improving the lot of those with a mental illness can exert influence. It also provides a legitimate means for carers to be able to express their views and perhaps even develop pressure group tactics, although such initiatives seem a long way away. These developments are very new, but they do provide limited grounds for optimism.

The influence of the China Federation of the Disabled is already visible in the matter of the *Eighth Five Year Plan for Disabled Persons 1991–1995*. Para 2:4 includes a specific provision for an experimental service delivery project for people with a mental illness. Thirty-two cities (urban) and 32 counties (rural) are to be selected for the provision of a comprehensive range of treatment and rehabilitation facilities on an experimental basis (Phillips & Pearson, 1994). A document circulated at the Second National Psychiatric Rehabilitation Meeting held in Chengdu in 1992, emanating from the China Federation for the Disabled, gave more details.

Among other things, this document recommends:

1. That the main coordination work be carried out by the local offices of the China Federation for the Disabled in conjunction with the representatives of the Departments of Public Security, Public Health and Civil Affairs.
2. That street level committees in the cities, townships and villages having more than 1000 inhabitants should form 'three man leading groups' and nominate someone to be responsible for daily work and planning.
3. Families of psychiatric patients should select a representative to liaise with the above groups.
4. Each province, autonomous region and Shanghai, Beijing and Tianjin will designate a mental health institution to be a training centre for all grades of staff. Emphasis will be given to community care and prevention.
5. At the county level in rural areas a mental health institution should be formed or designated to find patients currently not receiving treatment, keep a record of patients, undertake public education and provide treatment.
6. Guardianship networks should be set up. (These are discussed in more detail in Chapter 4.)
7. Domiciliary services should be provided for unstable patients who cannot be hospitalised.
8. All street level organisations, villages and towns should set up a work therapy station to provide some occupation, recreation and medical supervision. It is also suggested that psychiatric hospitals set up factories, work stations or farms to provide remunerated employment for those who are well enough to leave but have nowhere to go. Large factories and enterprises employing workers with a mental illness are recommended to set up work therapy stations as an integral part of their operations.

Two general principles are suggested. First, 'back to the community' should be the watchword for those who are stable or whose illness is not too severe. Second, 'don't lock patients up'. This refers not to hospitals, but to those patients who continue to be imprisoned at home by their families and whose existence is frequently a secret. This is more of a problem in rural areas where standards of education are lower and access to treatment much more difficult.

When this document was discussed at the Second National Psychiatric Rehabilitation Meeting in Chengdu in May 1992, the general consensus in the small discussion group in which I was placed was that the ideas contained in it were good. The problems identified were finance and the unsupportive attitude of cadres and the general public.

The document specified that central government funds would be very restricted, although the government has set aside about three million US dollars from central funds. The new services are supposed to be supported out of a local tax of five fen (which would buy half a small banana in the market) on each resident. In addition, individuals and organisations were to be asked to donate money, for instance, to support the work stations. Conference delegates were frankly disbelieving that this would work.

We find the same sort of problem in the official *Eighth Five Year Plan* which in paragraph 2:6 says that "local governments at all levels are requested to increase budgetary allocations to rehabilitation services". For as long as the central authorities lack the resources to contribute significant funds to these sorts of projects, they will lack the necessary clout to ensure that they are implemented. It seems likely that the '64-sites' project is going to founder on the rocky shores of inadequate financing and lack of local support. Where it is successful, it is likely that this will be due to a combination of circumstances. There will need to be individuals, who for some reason, are enthusiastic about the improvement of psychiatric services and who are also gifted with entrepreneurial skills. So far, it seems that this scheme has only taken off in areas where some, or all, of the suggested facilities and services were already in existence (Phillips & Pearson, 1994).

Conclusions

Whatever their views on China's political system, most Western observers assume that, as a socialist country, it will have health and welfare services (even if of a relatively low level) freely available to all citizens. The facts contradict such assumptions. Of particular surprise is the very high cost to the consumer of in-patient hospital treatment. A relatively small section of the population, urban workers in large or state owned enterprises, enjoys quite generous welfare benefits. However, the majority in effect have to fend for themselves.

The strategy emphasises the devolution and decentralisation of welfare responsibilities away from the state and towards the family, *danwei*, street organisation, and villages and townships. A motto of the Ministry of Civil Affairs is "self-reliance by the masses; mutual aid and dependency within the collective; state help as a last resort".

The rural–urban divide has bedevilled health policy in China since the beginning of the century. The difficulties of providing services to the rural population are, of course, shared with other countries with large rural areas. There is strong and deep-seated reluctance amongst Chinese physicians to work in the countryside. The resources needed to send doctors to train rural-based paramedics, or provide mobile clinics would be enormous. This is probably the most important issue facing the development of psychiatric services in China. The disparity between urban workers with health benefits and the rural population largely without has led to gross inequality in access to treatment.

One of the most significant issues that the People's Republic has to face in the provision of psychiatric care is that of sufficient, trained personnel, who are motivated to work in this area. Insufficient input on psychiatry at the level of basic training and the lack of a national programme of accreditation for postgraduates will continue to hamper professional development.

It seems that health care is less a priority now than at any other time since the founding of the People's Republic. Much has been achieved but there is no longer a sense of vision about the path that health care is taking, either in general health or in psychiatry. Hillier & Jewell (1983) talk about a policy of gradualism being no policy at all because it reacts to events rather than decides them. Many of the issues which face China's health policy makers are to do with structural aspects of society rather than individual health promoting habits and thus require change at the economic and political levels. These are not likely to be forthcoming. Most importantly, the issue of how services are financed is affecting accessibility to much needed care, and putting it beyond the reach of those who need it most. This is a strange irony in a socialist country.

4   The patient in the community

Various systems, both formal and informal, impinge upon the patient in the community, including the family, work place, the legal system and formal agencies such as street organisations and clinics. With the scarcity of hospital beds, many people with even a severe psychiatric disorder spend most, and frequently all, of their lives outside a hospital. The 1987 document on improving psychiatric care discussed in Chapter 3 claims that 85% of psychiatric patients cannot receive treatment and 95% of them cannot be admitted to psychiatric hospital.

Thus what happens to patients outside the hospital setting should be of considerable importance. Yet doctors tend to be very much more orientated towards bed-based care than any community-based alternative. One of the consequences of this is that the contribution of families to the care of people with a mental illness goes unrecognised. Of course, families carry the responsibility for caring everywhere, and it is only relatively recently that their contribution has been acknowledged in the UK and the USA (Perring *et al*, 1990). But whereas it is estimated that in the USA 40% of patients with schizophrenia are cared for by their families (Torrey, 1988), in China the figure is closer to 95% (Pearson & Phillips, 1994*a*). Thus families are overwhelmingly the most important resource in the care of patients.

In addition, the collective structures of the *danwei* and the street or neighbourhood organisation may also provide support. The role and function of the *danwei* have been discussed in Chapter 3. For someone who is unemployed, retired or a full-time homemaker, the street organisation performs many of the tasks of social and political integration and control normally carried out by the *danwei*. More information about the administrative structure of urban areas with regard to social welfare may be found in Wong

(1992). The street office operates on authority delegated from the district level of the city and, although not a government agency, wields considerable influence over its jurisdiction which may extend from 1200 to 5000 households. Many services are provided at this level, and include taking some responsibility for disabled people without a job living at home, including those with a mental illness.

Attitudes towards mental illness and mentally ill people

Any care offered to people with a mental illness living outside the hospital is going to be greatly affected by the attitude of others towards them. Consequently, it is necessary to have a sense of the social environment in which these tasks have to be undertaken.

Dear (1984) suggests that there are three major potential community attitudes towards people with a mental illness: authoritarianism, which implies a view of them as an inferior class needing coercive handling; benevolence, which embodies a paternalistic, kindly view of patients derived from humanistic and religious principles; and social restrictiveness, viewing the mentally ill as a threat to society. Elements of all three may be observed in the approach to community facilities for people with a mental illness in China. Such people are not necessarily seen as inferior, but as unable to control themselves and therefore in need of control by others. Benevolence, where it exists, is more likely to stem from a sense of shared political community and citizenship rather than religious or even humanistic principles.

The 1987 document *Opinions On Strengthening Mental Health Work* makes it clear that the government is deeply concerned with the capacity of mentally disordered people to cause social disruption. The major paradigm that guides policy initiatives at national or local level is concerned with controlling people with a mental illness and minimising their potential for creating social disorder. The preservation of individual freedoms is not an issue (Pearson, 1992*b*); this is entirely consistent with the official approach in China to other social and political issues.

Informal responses to mental illness

It is true that in Western countries, having a mentally ill person in the family is often a cause for deep concern. There are the practical difficulties that this poses, plus an awareness of the possibility of illness being passed on to future generations. The same sort of concern is experienced in China but at such a level of intensity as to make it not only different in degree but almost in kind.

To have a family member who is mentally ill is a matter of such intense shame that only in the most dire circumstances will it be made known to other than the closest of relatives, and not always then (Phillips, 1993). There is a widespread belief that mental illness is a punishment for the ancestors' misdeeds visited on the present generation, effectively shaming several generations of the family simultaneously. The 'taint' associated with mental illness is so strong that it extends beyond the affected person, for instance with regard to the issue of marriage. It might be expected that the patient's chances of finding a spouse would be affected but so are those of the siblings. On occasion, families split up and move to different areas, with one parent taking the ill child and the other one the siblings in order that the secret may be better kept and their siblings' chances of marriage unaffected.

In addition to this, 'madness' is associated with strange, violent and deviant acts in a society where conformity and reticence are highly valued. While those living in urban areas are familiar with the concept of mental disorder as an illness, in rural areas it is still very common to attribute mental illness to spirit possession (Li & Phillips, 1990; Pearson, 1993), further adding to the negative and fearful connotations. All in all, this adds up to a very unaccepting environment for people with a mental illness and their families. As reported in interviews with family members, there is no expectation of help or support from neighbours, only mockery at best and physical harm at worst.

These negative attitudes extend to the medical and nursing professions, because the staff are afraid of people with a mental illness. General hospital wards refuse to admit psychiatric patients who are suffering from a non-psychiatric illness and require treatment (Bueber, 1993a). Newly qualified doctors and nurses consider that they have been extraordinarily unlucky if they are allocated to the psychiatric field and make very reluctant recruits, further affecting the quality of care that can be offered. Some nurses are so untrusting of patients that they will not tell them their names and genuinely fear that they may 'catch' schizophrenia (Bueber, 1992b).

The contribution of the family

The family is required to take on its considerable responsibilities vis-a-vis a member with a mental illness in an environment which is essentially hostile. The government has been reluctant to do anything that would detract from the necessity for families to take care of their own, on the grounds that the resources needed would grossly exceed anything the government could reasonably provide (Wong, 1992). Furthermore, what services there are generally only apply to the urban areas. There are continuing and intractable difficulties in delivering even medication to mentally ill people in rural areas, let alone any other kind of service.

Lin (1984) argues that the reluctance of the government to intervene in the care of people with a mental illness is compounded by the nature of mental disorder as a taboo area, and the unwillingness of lay people or the authorities to face the issue squarely. This has led to an over-reliance on the traditional family centred approach.

China is a family orientated country. We need, however, to have a clearer idea of what that means, and how the microcosm of the family links into a wider social network and expectations of relationships.

The individual, the family and society

Yang (1986) sums up the personality characteristics of the Chinese as being socially orientated with collectivistic, authoritarian tendencies, and a submissive and inhibited disposition. He relates these characteristics to a predominantly agricultural subsistence economy that lasted for millennia; to a social structure that is hierarchical, collectivist, structurally tight and based on what he calls generalised familisation; and to patterns of socialisation which emphasise dependency, conformity, modesty, self-suppression, and parent-centredness. He also sees signs of change.

Hsu (1985), in a thesis famous in cross-cultural psychology, suggests that the concept of personality, as an expression of individualism, is not applicable to the Chinese. He posits a model that sees man, culture and society as a series of concentric circles. The innermost circles represent the unconscious and pre-conscious; the next two the inexpressible and expressible conscious, surrounded by intimate society and culture, operative society and culture, wider society and culture; and finally the outer world. This system he calls psychodynamic homeostasis (PSH) represented by the Confucian concept of *ren* (variously translated as 'benevolence', 'human heartedness' and 'humanity'). One of the effects of this is that the Western impetus for children and young adults to achieve independence from their parents is not found in China. The culturally valued position is that there will be a life-long mutual dependence between parents and children, where the balance in care-giving changes gradually as both parties age.

In some ways Hsu was ahead of the field, for he formulated his ideas at a time in Western psychology, the 1960s and 1970s, when the concept of personality tended to be construed as a static given, constant in many different situations and with many different people. His interactionist, flexible notion of the individual in relation to others, behaving differently in different contexts has been adopted by main stream Western psychology as a more fruitful way of looking at all human beings.

One of Hsu's fundamental theses is that Chinese people do not have to go beyond the family to satisfy their intimacy needs, and that attachment to parents provides a stability and continuity that is lacking in Western people's search for intimate relations. He goes on to suggest that his PSH layer of intimate society and culture are not the same in Chinese/Japanese as opposed to Western cultures. The former are characterised by more ritualisation, role playing, hierarchical relationships and repression of negativity, repression of personal spontaneity when compared with Western ideals. These factors make it more difficult for intimacy as Westerners think of it to occur. Family stability and security are maintained at the cost of the Western concepts of intimacy and independence. But this is because the Chinese and Japanese are not seeking a conceptually equivalent type of intimacy. The stability and reliability of intimate relationships with others are a source of strength for the individual and the society. The question is how and whether different cultures provide for this need, and the tolerances and implications for differences in the experience of need.

Confucianism

"A child in China is born into a family and placed in a network of inter-related persons. The self does not develop in a process of gradual separation and individuation as is often conceptualised in Western psychological theories. We see instead a 'little me' maintaining its interdependency within the context of the 'big me' the family, the state and the world throughout the philosophical traditions of Confucianism and Taoism as well as present day socialist theory." (Dien, 1983, p.284)

King & Bond (1985) argue that while Confucianism as a social theory tends to mould the Chinese into group and family orientated, socially dependent beings, it also represents only part of the total complexity. The Confucian thrust is also to develop a person into a relation orientated individual who is capable of asserting a self-directed role in constructing a social world. If this was not so it would make a nonsense of Confucius' ideal of a righteous man, who achieved this condition through self-cultivation, nurturing the values of *ren*, and being able to recognise what was morally correct and do it.

Confucius was writing at a time of great social upheaval and this may account for the emphasis he places on harmony as the most treasured social value. He argues that harmony may only be achieved by everyone acting towards others in a proper way. The proper way is defined by the rules of propriety (*li*). This defines correct behaviour in a series of social relationships that will maintain harmony for as long as each person acts according to the rules. According to Lin: "In the Chinese view, a person is a relational being, living and interacting in a massively complicated role system" (Lin, 1983, p. 866).

The maintenance of harmony is so important that it takes precedence over the expression of one's own opinions or feelings. As many authors point out, external compliance should not be mistaken for internal acceptance (King & Bond, 1985; Yang, 1986; Pye, 1988). The ability to adjust oneself to the situation is greatly valued over the idea that the situation should adjust to you.

Most social relationships are seen in hierarchical terms, expressed by the Five Cardinal Relationships, the *wu lun*; the Emperor and his subjects, father and son, older brother and younger brother, husband and wife, and friends. Only the last of these is based on anything like equal footing and even then friendships tend to be interpreted in terms of kinship relations, so almost inevitably friendships take on a hierarchical component, one or other of the pair tends to be the 'big brother' or 'big sister'.

The most important relationship within the family is that between father and son, or, more generally, between parents and children. The marital relationship is less significant and even now is frequently based on an alliance of interests rather than mutual affection. Hierarchies in the family are based on age, sex and generational position. Outside it, they are also based on status (Baker, 1979; King & Bond, 1985). Filial piety is an extension of this authority within the family and beyond to the individual's relation with the state.

The Communist Party's initial desire was to rid people of Confucian thinking, seeing it in fundamental opposition to their own philosophy and as a potential rival to their own political control. Over the years, however, they came to realise (as the Mandarinate had done before them), that there was much about the structure (if not the content) of social relationships guided by Confucianism that was not only congruent with their own, but useful to them. The reliance on higher authorities, the emphasis on obedience and acceptance of hierarchies and ultimately the ability of the family to control and order its members made China governable for millennia. And it does so still.

Family values

There are some fundamental differences in the way that Chinese and Western people view the family. To a modern Westerner, families might well be seen as a mixed blessing; nurturing but restrictive, hampering freedom and independence. This perspective is rarely aired in public by Chinese people, although clinical experience suggests that family conflicts abound. When one considers the poor and cramped living conditions, frequent lack of privacy (with two or three generations living in one room) and various other factors, it is not surprising that reality does not live up to the image. Here, two contrasting views are offered:

> "For Chinese people, the importance of the family, the institution which has patterned the entire social matrix can hardly be over-estimated. It is the bastion of their personal and economic security; it provides the frame of reference for personal and social organization; it controls all the behavioural and human relationships of its members through a clearly hierarchical structure and sanctioned mode of conduct; it transmits moral, religious and social values from generation to generation through role modelling, coercion and discipline. It offers a haven for safety, rest and recreation. The influence of the family on the lives of its mentally ill is no less profound than it is for anyone else." (Lin & Lin, 1981, p. 387)

> "The family, with its friends, became a walled castle with the greatest communistic co-operation and mutual help within but coldly indifferent toward and fortified against the world without. In the end, as it worked out, the family became a walled castle

outside which everything is legitimate loot". (Lin Yu Tang, 1935, quoted in Bodde, 1957, p. 67)

The obligation to care

Westerners tend to admire the reliance on family care seen in China. It reminds them of that mythical period, much beloved of the New Right, when 'community care' naturally occurred and did not have to be planned by governments. But such admiration fails to take into account the stress and burden that Chinese families suffer in much the same way as their Western counterparts.

Based on their work in the Chinese community in Vancouver, Lin & Lin (1981) have identified five stages of familial coping with mental illness:

1. Exclusively intrafamilial coping
2. Inclusion of certain trusted outsiders in the intrafamilial attempt at coping
3. Consultation with outside helping agencies, physicians and finally a psychiatrist while keeping the patient at home
4. Labelling of mental illness and subsequent series of hospitalisations
5. Scapegoating and rejection.

They say that the first three stages are characterised by 'tender loving care', protection and intense efforts to mobilise helping resources. Once the mental illness has been labelled, a radical change in family attitude seems to take place, and the family becomes less tolerant. Their guilt, frustration, fear and anger are directed at the patient and the tender loving care is replaced with tension, worry and desperation.

It is difficult to know whether or not this schema is typical of family reactions in China. If the onset of mental illness is florid and sudden, the family may be given little choice but to seek outside help, as other members of the community may not be prepared to tolerate such behaviour. The potential for rejection in such a tightly knit, geographically immobile and poorly resourced country is limited. The likelihood is that for many families the caring role is one they adopt out of a sense of affection and responsibility. For some, it may be because there is no alternative. There is no way to know how the relative proportions are distributed between these two positions. It is noteworthy that the 1980 Marriage Law lays down the duty of the different generations to care for each other in Articles 14, 15, and

22 suggesting that the obligation to care needs to be formally reinforced.

What is known is that the decision to seek treatment, what kind of treatment, and the amount of money to be spent on it, are all family decisions over which the patient has little or no control (Pearson & Phillips, 1994*b*). Once accepted as mentally ill, the person is considered unable to have a lucid opinion about their situation. Family members will accompany patients to the hospital on most occasions and frequently stay with them once admitted. This is also seen in medical hospitals (Henderson & Cohen, 1984).

The goals of caring

Coming to terms with schizophrenia, particularly if the patient is a young person, is a potentially lengthy task for the family. Every remission and every relapse contributes to an emotional roller coaster as the family continue to hope for a cure and search for different types of treatment. The more hopes had been invested in the patient for the improvement of the family future, the greater the sense of loss and mourning (Phillips, 1993). The situation is made even more poignant because of the effects of the government's 'one-child' policy, particularly in the urban areas. Increasingly, the mentally ill child will be the only child of the family.

Once the family have come to terms with the nature of the illness, their strategies are likely to be aimed at ensuring the patient's (and to some extent their own) future security. It must be remembered that there are no intermediaries, such as social workers, to help them find a path through the maze (Pearson & Phillips, 1994*a*). They can use only their own resources and *guanxi* (connections). In life, three things need to be achieved: a spouse, a child and a job (Phillips, 1993).

A spouse

China is very much a couple orientated society and being unmarried is a stigma. Parents generally take a distinctly proactive stance in the search for a spouse. Arranged marriages are not uncommon, especially in the rural areas. However, the level of fear of mental illness is such that frequently the illness is hidden from the potential spouse, or some kind of trade-off is agreed. In interviewing patients and relatives I came across several examples of this. The most common is that a person from a rural area will agree to marry a mentally ill person with an urban *hukou* (residence permit). This then gives them the right to live in the city, an opportunity much treasured. Or it may be that someone else who is considered 'damaged goods' will be found as a spouse, for instance, a women with epilepsy who agrees to marry a man with schizophrenia. The parents of the mentally ill person, whether it be a son or a daughter, are likely to continue to take a lively interest in the marriage.

A child

Obviously, unless the parents can ensure a marriage, they live with the spectre of who will take care of the patient once they are dead. This is at least partly the reason why a child is considered important, despite the official strictures against people with schizophrenia having children (see also Chapter 2). In a marriage where the affectional bonds are not considered strong, it is thought that a child will bind the couple together. Although still very low, the divorce rate among people with schizophrenia is ten times that of the general population: 6.5% and 0.67% respectively (Phillips, 1993). In addition, there is the traditional and still very strong desire for a grandchild, preferably a grandson. A child also provides someone to care for both older generations as they age.

The long-term effects of China's 'one child' policy should not be overlooked in this regard. Concern has been widely expressed in China about the burden that will befall only children looking after two sets of parents/in-laws. The added dimension of a mentally ill parent who is not able to assume responsibility for the grandparent generation will compound the problem. From the parents' point of view, the lack of siblings will constrict even further the range of caring possibilities for a child with mental illness.

A job

Employment is often a contributing factor to continued mental health, normalisation and sense of self-worth (Wansborough, 1981; Watts & Bennett, 1991). In China, not only are these more individualistic concerns important, but there is also the societal imperative of contributing to the construction of socialism through labour. To be without employment is to be severely disadvantaged, not only economically but socially and politically.

Finding a job is much more an issue for those living in the urban areas. Patients from the rural areas will almost certainly be able to perform some agricultural tasks on the family farm, although there may be costs to the family in that the patient may not be able to perform at the expected level, thus reducing the family income. The situation for patients in the urban areas is concentrated upon here.

Chinese citizens, until comparatively recently, enjoyed a job for life – 'the iron rice bowl'. It may not have been a job they liked, and certainly not one they chose, but they could rely on being given a job when they left school that would be theirs for ever. Along with the job came a *danwei* and through it, access to the range of welfare benefits that were outlined in Chapter 3. Enterprises, factories, government departments were supported by the state, however bloated their work force. If they made a profit, that was appreciated, but if not, it was not a major issue. Wages and bonuses would still be forthcoming.

This situation has been changing over the last decade with the introduction of the 'socialist commodity economy' (which, to an outsider, looks remarkably like capitalism). This has had a serious effect on the employability of people with a mental illness (Pearson, 1989). Under previous conditions it did not matter whether or not they were slower than their work mates, or if they needed to take more sick leave. Now that bonuses are related to performance, managers are extremely reluctant to employ someone who has a history of mental illness and fellow employees are unwilling to work with them.

For older people, already in employment under the old conditions, the situation is not so bad, although they may be made to feel unwelcome and even paid a reduced salary and asked to stay at home. But for youngsters trying to enter the job market, the situation is very difficult indeed.

It is increasingly rare for a worker to be taken on 'for life'. Rather they are offered a contract first, usually for about three years. It is almost impossible for the family to hide the fact of the young employee's mental illness for that length of time, and once it becomes apparent, employment will be terminated, either at the end of the contract or immediately. Not only does this deprive the family of one of its sources of income but it also means that the patient is no longer covered by health insurance, and the family are therefore liable for the considerable costs incurred by any future admissions. The cumulative effect of this is that as the years pass, fewer and fewer people with a mental illness are going to be covered by health insurance because few of them will have jobs.

The strategies available to parents in this situation are limited. They are forced into using their own *guanxi* to the fullest extent in the search for some kind of employment for their child. This may involve using their influence at their own place of work, enrolling the assistance of relatives and friends, or bribing well-placed officials. With the introduction of a more open economy, there are more opportunities for people to establish their own businesses. Typically, these might include repair services for household goods (China is not a throw-away society) or running a small shop or street stall. But such activities provide neither security nor health insurance.

Helping systems

The help that families receive depends on two factors. First, different understandings of what causes psychiatric illness will lead to families seeking out different types of care. Second, their choice is restricted by what is available within what they consider to be reasonable travelling distance from their homes.

Chinese medicine is well known for its 'syncretism' (Kleinman, 1986), and Chinese people for their willingness to combine a variety of treatment approaches in a search for a cure or relief from suffering. Lin & Lin (1981) offer a five-category model for explanations of mental illness used by Chinese people, based on work in Taiwan and among Chinese communities in Canada. These are the moral view, the religious or cosmological view, physiological or medical theories, psychosocial factors and genetic transmission.

In a series of interviews carried out in an out-patients' department attached to a psychiatric hospital in Hubei province, it was found that families were most likely to seek explanations for their family members' illnesses in personality (78.3%), social (75.6%), supernatural (40.5%) and somatic (18.9%) factors. This was in contra-distinction to doctors who used primarily biological systems of explanation and showed little interest in psychosocial factors (Pearson, 1993).

Families saw no contradiction in seeking help from a Western trained doctor, a practitioner of Chinese traditional medicine and a ritual specialist during the same course of illness (Pearson, 1993). Sometimes this was because there was disagreement within the family, especially between older and younger members, as to the best strategy to adopt. At other times, it was because the family felt that it was their duty to do everything within their power to ensure the sick person's health. Occasionally, it was a case of 'if one thing does not work, try something else'.

Support for the family

As families provide most of the physical, emotional and social care for patients, it would seem that supporting and improving their attempts to do this would be an efficient use of scarce resources. Unfortunately, such approaches are, as yet, very limited. Two have been reported in the literature.

Zhang, Wang *et al* (1994) randomly assigned 78 male patients with a diagnosis of schizophrenia to a treatment or control group. Both treatment and control groups received standard medication but the treatment group also included individual and group counselling of family members. Subjects touched upon in the counselling sessions included: information about the illness; life events that occurred before and after the patient fell ill, and methods of avoiding or resolving these stressful circumstances; family members' attitudes towards the patient's illness; the importance of thinking about the patient's symptoms as manifestations of a 'bad personality' or fate; the necessity of not reprimanding the patient in a hostile manner; and the value of not being so over-concerned that one excessively restricts the patient's contact with the outside world. There was a significantly lower rate of rehospitalisation in the 18-month follow-up period in the family intervention group and the mean rehospitalisation-free period for those who were rehospitalised was significantly longer for those in the treatment group.

Interesting work is being produced by Phillips & Xiong in Hubei province (Xiong *et al*, in press). They have been working to develop a comprehensive, on-going intervention that is both suitable and feasible for most urban families of patients with schizophrenia, given the constraints of the Chinese mental health care system.

Intervention, aimed at those who meet DSM–III–R diagnostic criteria for schizophrenia, and their families, includes a two to three-month introductory phase, a one to two-year treatment phase and an on-going maintenance programme. It is based on regular 45-minute counselling sessions for patients and family members, that includes medication management, family education, behavioural treatment of patients' inappropriate behaviours, communication skills training, crisis intervention, and detailed discussion of social and occupational problems. Families and patients are also encouraged to attend a monthly support group meeting, and where necessary receive home visits, contact with employers and interviews with extended family members. At 6, 12 and 18 month follow-ups with evaluators blind to the groupings, the proportion of subjects rehospitalised in the treatment group was lower, the mean duration of rehospitalisation was shorter, and the duration of employment was longer.

Family intervention approaches

Varying approaches to family intervention have been developed in Western countries (Falloon *et al*, 1985; Tarrier *et al*, 1988; Leff *et al*, 1989) but all of them share three common elements (Shepherd, 1991). All aim to give family members more information about schizophrenia, aetiology, outcome, course and so on. Particularly important is the understanding that negative symptoms are symptoms rather than personal failings, and helping families to cope in a non-critical, non-judgemental way. Second, all approaches aim at improving communication and problem-solving skills. Thirdly, all programmes contain an element of non-specific emotional support. The two programmes described here also have those elements in common.

A more indigenous form of helping relatives is via a guardianship network (sometimes known as a psychiatric care unit). The *Eighth Five Year Plan For Disabled People* as it applies to those with a mental illness (see Chapter 3) describes these in some detail. At the moment only relatively few areas have adopted them (Shanghai, Guangzhou, Nanjing, Suzhou, for instance), but the document suggests that they should be made part of the national platform of services available for people with a mental illness.

Guardianship networks are to comprise residents' committee cadres, paramedical staff and the patients' family members. Their duties are as follows: visiting regularly, recording the patient's illness status, offering instructions about treatment and rehabilitation, mediating conflicts, solving problems, supervising patients to take medicine regularly, preventing self-harm or violence to others, or damage to property. Each police station should have close co-operation with the guardianship networks in its area to assist in managing the patient.

Descriptions of the current operation of these units are provided in Xia *et al* (1987), Pearson (1992*a*) and Qiu & Lu (1994). All of them emphasise the social control aspect of the guardianship network function. For instance, I was told in Beijing by a Department of Civil Affairs official that they were supposed to make sure that people with a mental illness were kept off the streets, stayed safely at home and took their medication. Some needed to be locked in. If possible, some sort of occupation is supposed to be provided at home. Most Western statements about looking after patients outside the hospital are couched in terms of what will provide the most normal living conditions for patients, increase their sense of self-worth and value and improve the quality of their lives. This is not an issue in China. The major concern is how to stop the collective being disturbed by the individual.

In practice, much of the day-to-day responsibility rests on the shoulders of the family member, as it would do in any case. Possibly, the benefit from their point of view is that with the existence of an official network, they are linked into others who have a recognised responsibility should they need guidance, face difficulties, or find that the patient starts to relapse.

Work-orientated interventions

We have already noted the philosophical, political and practical importance of work as part of the care of mentally ill people. Although mixed disability sheltered workshops exist, these, on the whole, will not accept people with a mental illness because of the negative attitude towards this group shared by both workers and staff. At a more local level, work therapy stations are provided. These are usually run by the Department of Civil Affairs or by street organisations. These small units cater for people with a variety of disabilities and do not exclude the mentally ill (Pearson, 1992*a*). Along with the guardianship networks, these form another fundamental plank in the strategy of the Eighth Five Year Plan for the care of people with a mental illness. Currently, the major centres like Beijing, Guangzhou, Nanjing and Shanghai have work stations, but their distribution elsewhere is unknown (Pearson 1992*a*; Luo & Yu, 1994; Zhang *et al*, 1994).

The quality and facilities of work stations vary. They all aim at providing some daily structure and purpose, by getting people out of their homes and providing them with a variety of activities. These may include some low-grade manufacturing work, educational, and recreational activities. Many of the workers are content to be there. Universally, in the seven or eight work stations I have visited in both Guangzhou and Beijing, it was said that the family members found the work stations a great blessing. Staffing is variable. It might consist of retired workers, perhaps a nurse, doctor or teacher, or it could be in the hands of junior Department of Civil Affairs staff with no relevant experience. Occasionally, staff will also have a disability (usually a physical one). Perhaps the recruitment of staff with disabilities is due to the link with the Department of Civil Affairs, one of whose many responsibilities is to find work for the disabled. A more thorough description of the structure and running of a work station is provided in Pearson (1992a).

Another alternative is to base services for people with a mental illness in factories, particularly the larger ones. Many factories provide medical services for their staff and dependents, including a clinic and even a small hospital on occasion. This is entirely consistent with Chinese expectations concerning the role of the work place in providing a wide range of health and welfare services.

In an article purporting to describe community psychiatry in China, Jiang (1988) says that if the factory is large enough, it will form a supervisory team consisting of the factory director and supervisory personnel from the trade union and the factory hospital. A mental health group is formed under its leadership for prevention and treatment throughout the factory. This group is also responsible for visiting families and forming guardianship networks. Their aim is to help those with a chronic mental illness recover their working ability and resume production. Lu (1978) and Pearson (1992a) both report on liaison schemes between psychiatric hospitals and large factories, where doctors from the hospital went to visit the factories to train clinic staff in a deeper understanding of psychiatric illness and to run public education programmes for workers, in the hope of increasing their tolerance and understanding of workmates with a mental illness.

More recently, another project has been reported in Nanjing (Luo & Yu, 1994), where seven large enterprises have organised their own sheltered workshops/work stations within the factory. These provide the same range of services as work stations located in a neighbourhood. They describe how the project first started in 1977. Factory leaders wanted to keep workers with a mental illness hospitalised for prolonged periods as a means of ensuring the security and tranquillity of the work place. However, family members were not willing to allow recovered patients to remain in hospital indefinitely. Nor were hospitals, at that time, willing to have their beds used in that way. Under these circumstances, patients returned home and were given full pay, but asked to stay away from work because the factory leaders were concerned that they would cause trouble. As Luo & Yu point out, this method of managing patients was detrimental to both patients and factory. Work stations in factories were then established. Luo & Yu's study of the outcome of this form of care found that the relapse and rehospitalisation rates were significantly higher in the control group than in the experimental treatment group.

This model has been developed as one which is indigenous to China and takes account of the cultural imperatives in operation there. It is worth noting, however, that this report records that the patients were sometimes resistant to going to the work station, preferring to move straight back into the factory because they could earn more there. One cannot help but wonder whether some of their reluctance might be based on a sense of the stigmatisng nature of the work station, which publicly labels them as psychiatrically disabled, if only temporarily.

A model project is run by Dr Wang Xishi in Shenyang city in Liaoning Province (Pearson, 1992*a*; Wang, 1994). Originally, in 1975, the Department of Civil Affairs set up a 'prevention and cure psychiatric centre' in response to concerns about patients who could not control their behaviour and who adversely affected social stability (*China Civil Affairs*, No. 9, September 1987). Through a combination of clinical and entrepreneurial skills, Dr Wang has managed to finance a comprehensive psychiatric service (including a 65-bedded hospital, an out-patients' department and a domicilliary service) on the basis of a factory that prints cinema tickets. Fifty-one per cent of the workforce are ex-psychiatric patients. This project demonstrates that within the Chinese system there is room for change and innovation. Sadly, it has not been replicated elsewhere.

Why no accommodation alternatives?

One familiar service missing from the social services outlined so far is non-family accommodation outside of hospital. The vast majority of people live with family members. Yet in any large city, there will be a number of patients who have no one willing to take responsibility for them. Even in acute hospitals there will be a number of patients who have been there for over a year because they have nowhere else to go. My experience of the Municipal Hospital was that a significant number of patients were sufficiently stable to be discharged but no one wanted them. Indeed chronicity, in some cases, seemed to be a function of social deprivation in this regard rather than of symptomatology. So why have accommodation alternatives not developed?

The most obvious reason is that it is against the family ethos. There is a strong feeling on the part of individuals that it is their right to be cared for within a family context. Not to be so cared for is stigmatising in itself. Secondly, from the point of view of officials, the financial consequences of accepting responsibility for housing mentally ill persons would be frightening. Further, as one psychiatrist from Shanghai pointed out, the government has a chronic housing shortage in the large cities. The general public would resent resources being used to house mentally ill people when 'normal' people do not have a decent place to live. In addition, the general consensus among psychiatrists with whom I have discussed this matter is that the man in the street would not accept independently housed mentally ill people as neighbours. Attempts to provide housing for them might lead to social unrest.

In structural terms, the provision of housing would cut across pre-existing administrative responsibilities. Outside the hospital, a person with a mental illness is not the responsibility of anyone by virtue simply of his or her illness. He is the family's responsibility because of blood ties; responsibility of the *danwei* because he is a worker; and the neighbourhood's responsibility because he lives there. There is no collective organisation based in the community that is responsible for looking after people with a mental illness. *Danweis* do not have enough people with a mental illness to provoke them into the search for alternative housing; the same is true of neighbourhoods. In both cases, there would need to be some way of generating the necessary finance to cover costs or even make a profit and this is unlikely to occur. At the collective levels at which services are currently provided, it is not enough of a problem to motivate people to search for a solution.

Medical services

If this is the position with regard to social services for people with a mental illness, what of community-based health services? On the whole, such services are scarce. Psychiatric hospitals in towns and cities usually include an out-patients' department. Day hospitals are not widely reported in the literature, although a mention of their existence in Shanghai is made by Zhang, Yan *et al* (1994), and a day hospital has recently opened in Wuhan. There are no crisis intervention services and families who want to have someone admitted must find a way to get them to the hospital by themselves or, if the situation is sufficiently difficult, involve the police.

Some families consult a doctor at a general clinic but many simply make the decision themselves that the patient needs to be admitted. Where they are taken depends on the level of knowledge of the family and the facilities available. Many families subvert the 'referring-up' system, whereby smaller, local and less well-staffed facilities are supposed to filter out the less serious cases and refer the more difficult ones to a hospital of a higher standard. Families tend to take the patient to the best hospital they can afford, if there is a choice.

The interviewing doctor in the out-patients department therefore has no referral letter or background information about the patient. There is no system whereby a patient attending more than once can see the same doctor. This means that the patient and family must tell their story afresh every time they visit – if the doctor is willing to listen – as records on out-patients are not kept. Interviews are cursory and usually last less than ten minutes. If they forget to bring the small piece of paper they are given on which the prescribed medication is recorded, the medical staff have no idea what previous medication was prescribed or what the original diagnosis was. In the acute hospital in Hubei with which I am most familiar, the ward doctors do not take out-patients clinics, so it is impossible for them to follow up patients on discharge. Nor is there any method of referring a patient on discharge to a doctor nearer his home for those who live outside of town. Patients and families must come back to the hospital for further supplies of medication. The inconvenience of this may contribute to the temptation to cease taking it – invariably the most common reason cited by doctors for patients suffering a relapse. My observations are confirmed by Zhang, Wang *et al* (1994) in their description of standard care in an out-patients department in Suzhou.

The only addition to the out-patients department which may be found in some areas are 'home beds' (Pearson, 1992*a*). Mention of home beds in China was first made by Wu (1959), where it was reported that the authorities in Nanjing had established 200 'sick beds' in the homes of psychiatric patients. Essentially, these are domicilliary services provided by mental health workers for discharged patients who are not well enough to attend an out-patients department or work on a regular basis, and yet do not need full hospital care. In the UK the closest comparison is probably the community psychiatric nursing service. Home beds have been used in Beijing (Shen, 1983, 1985) but the project there is relatively small, and Zhang, Wang *et al* (1994) report that Suzhou has 400 home beds.

Delivering services to rural areas is very difficult. On paper, there is a system of health organisation that reaches from towns and counties through townships to village clinics. Pearson (1995) provides a more detailed analysis of the structure. This system should permit psychiatric health delivery down to the village level. Unfortunately, the organisational and political will to make it work is frequently lacking. Only in two areas am I aware that this works as it is supposed to and, not surprisingly, both are acknowledged as model projects, not only in China but internationally.

The first of these is in Shandong province, based in the city of Yantai (Yao, 1985; Wang *et al*, 1994), which has attracted the interest of the World Health Organization and the World Association for Psychosocial Rehabilitation. The second, supported by the China Medical Board, is in Sichuan province, in Xinjin district outside Chengdu. This has not yet been written up in the English language literature. However, both work on similar principles, consisting of a three-tier network at county, township and village level. Training in psychiatry is provided to non-psychiatric doctors at both the township and village levels by psychiatrists from the 'mother' psychiatric hospital at county level. The village and township doctors work to establish a psychiatric register in their area and to set up 'home beds' for people with a mental disorder so that they are regularly visited and receive medication. In Yantai, 8000 home beds have been established since the beginning of the programme in 1977. In 1990, 3347 patients were enrolled, 85% of whom suffered from schizophrenia (Wang *et al*, 1994). They report that there is a marked decrease in dangerous behaviour and relapses, while there is an equally obvious increase in the number able to do full or part-time work.

Setting up such a service is a task of great complexity. The three major departments always involved in psychiatric care have to be co-ordinated at the three different levels. Apart from anything else, that means finding a large number of people who are sufficiently enthusiastic about the project to put time and effort into overcoming the many obstacles, and who can work together. Then there is the question of finance. The Yantai project is particularly remarkable in this respect, having been largely locally financed from its inception. This means that choices were made to channel money towards helping people with a mental illness, rather than some other more popular or 'glamorous' cause. Although a remarkable project, it is not one that has been easy for other areas in China to replicate, despite it being a home-grown model.

Do patients and families get what they want?

Few people have thought to ask this question. In a small scale study I undertook (Pearson & Jin, 1992) a small sample (n = 18) of relatives were interviewed and among other things were asked about their expectations of the encounter with the psychiatric hospital and whether they were satisfied. It has to be borne in mind that their experience of services was limited and they were not in a position to know the full range of alternatives. Their expectations of the doctors were quite clear. They expected doctors to make the patient well again and to the extent that this happened they were more or less satisfied. They expected doctors to be directive and authoritative and were willing to rely on their expert knowledge. What troubled them most was the lack of information they were given about the diagnosis, treatment and management of the patient. From observation of doctors' interviewing style, it was very clear that they did not see relatives as partners in care. They were reluctant to share information with them and were brusque and interrogative.

Perring *et al* (1990), in a review of the literature concerning the carers of people with a mental illness, list the needs of relatives as: information and involvement, support in a crisis, respite and day care, advice on how to manage difficult behaviour, advice on welfare benefits, and help with transport. Kuipers (1991) adds continuity, trust and understanding in the relationship with professionals. Although it cannot be assumed that relatives in the West have the same needs as those in China, it is likely that the similarity in experience of caring for someone with a psychotic disorder means that their needs would follow roughly similar directions. If a patient in China was fortunate enough to live in an area where Phillips (1993) or Zhang, Wang *et al* (1994) were practising, then many of these relatives' needs might be met. Some carers benefit from the day care provided by work stations. But on the whole, many of these needs go unmet.

Kuipers (1991) lists the needs of patients as: support, the provision of day care activity and structure, fostering independence, development and maintenance of self-help skills, practical help, physical care and individual counselling. If we know little about what relatives of patients want, we know even less about what the patients themselves think they need. An educated guess would suggest that support and daytime activity would probably be relevant to them. Fostering independence probably would not, although advice on how to manage intense family relationships in crowded conditions probably would (Pearson & Phillips, 1994a). It will be a long time, if ever, before we see an empowerment and advocacy movement among psychiatric patients and their relatives in China. As far as is known, only two support groups for relatives and patients have been established. One is in Shanghai and the other in Shashi (Hubei province) and both concentrate on providing support, education and recreation. The *Eighth Five Year Plan for the Disabled* envisions a greater role for relatives through the local branches of the All China Federation for the Disabled. Theoretically, if families exerted sufficient pressure on the government via this route, it might provoke it into doing more. But this seems unlikely.

Conclusions

The intention behind the provision of services in the community is very much one of maintaining social order. The Public Security arm of the government at both national and local levels is thus routinely involved with the provision of services and the supervision of patients. The goal is twofold: to ensure that the mentally ill do not cause trouble and to attempt to find them a productive role so that they can contribute to society. Whereas in Western countries the emphasis is on the self-acualisation and independence of the individual patient, in China the needs of society are given more prominence and the patient is expected to fit around them.

The major burden of care falls to the family, but for most families there is little or no outside help in negotiating with various systems to achieve the goals they seek for themselves and the patient. There are no social workers to assist with liaison functions, no non-governmental agencies to whom they can turn for ancillary aid. Furthermore, their considerable contribution as a caring resource is largely overlooked or taken for granted. Supporting and strengthening the family in its efforts to care is not seen as a relevant task for the medical services.

There is a clearly articulated model of community based care for the psychiatrically ill in China relying on work stations, guardianship networks, factory based services and 'home beds', but implementing it is very problematic (Pearson, 1992a). The central authorities have insufficient power and money to impose their definition of a good service on the provinces, leaving local development to the enthusiasm and good will of local people. The end result is that change is slow and that outside major centres there is little support for families.

This then raises the question of whether, as they become wealthier and are able to purchase alternatives, families will continue to care for their mentally ill family members at home. At the moment, most do not have a choice, but, already, small, private institutions are springing up offering cheaper prices than standard hospital care. Facilities are basic at best and staff are frequently untrained. There is no system of registration. They are developing, however, because families are willing to use them and because the owners can make a profit.

It is likely that many families in China would prefer to shift the burden of caring elsewhere, given the choice. This is, at least partly, a consequence of the authorities' expectation that patients will shape themselves to the services, rather than providing patients and their relatives with services which meet their needs. Unless Chinese mental health policy begins seriously to focus on the family as a resource to be preserved and strengthened, the move in the future will be towards increased institutionalisation.

Another feature of the system that will fuel the shift towards the provision of more hospital beds and away from community based services is the increasing demand from the government that hospitals be more and more self-financing. With this move comes the raising of fees for in-patient care as the easiest source of funds. At the moment, however, a number of the 'home bed' schemes are dependent on hospitals to provide supervisory staff, training to lower grade staff and various other support services. Hospitals may decide that they can no longer afford the time that providing such help takes away from fee-generating activities. An even more fundamental problem is that the more success models like the Yantai project enjoy, the less need there will be for hospitals. Thus any hospital helping such a project will in the long term be reducing the demand for in-patient care and shrinking its income in the process. All in all, the future for care in the community of psychiatric patients does not look promising.

5   The Municipal Hospital

I first made contact with the Municipal Hospital in 1987, and the attitude of the Medical Superintendent encouraged me to broach the possibility of research. Clearly, the Medical Superintendent was interested and personally willing to participate. However, much negotiation within the labyrinthine byways of the Chinese bureaucracy was needed before permission was eventually granted. The visits to the hospital took place over the summer and autumn of 1988, when most of the empirical data was collected, and regular contact has been maintained since.

There is no way to tell how typical the Municipal Hospital is of psychiatric hospitals in China generally. It is not the best but it is certainly not the worst. Conditions there are infinitely better than those reported by Western journalists in Heilongjiang and Tianjin ('The Asylums of China': The *Independent* Magazine, 11 March 1990) and in Dali Psychiatric Hospital in Yunnan province ('In Search of a Sane Society': *South China Morning Post*, 19 November 1988). The hospital has received very few foreign guests and it is certainly not one of those hospitals chosen to be shown to foreigners.

Those Western writers who have lived in China or who have had more extensive experience of Chinese conditions (Yan *et al*, 1984; Kleinman, 1986; Altschuler *et al*, 1988; Phillips, 1993) are all doctors or, in the case of Bueber, a nurse (1992, 1993*a,b,c*; Bueber *et al*, 1993). Consequently, they tend not to write about the management of hospitals and psychiatric resources generally, but are largely concerned with issues of diagnosis and treatment, leaving something of a gap in our knowledge. The material gathered at the Municipal Hospital offers a new perspective on our current understanding of psychiatric care in China.

I was permitted to spend one month at the hospital and given relatively free access to areas over which the Medical Superintendent had control. These included patients' files, staff and patients themselves. I was permitted to run an essay competition for patients as part of the research, and found myself awarding prizes after recreational activities and taking part in other public events involving patients. It was not possible to contact patients' relatives. From the patients' viewpoint, my visits to wards were a welcome diversion. There were always some who wanted to practise their English and many who would gather round firing questions at me about where I came from, what I did, was I married and so on.

On the whole, staff were friendly and co-operative, although somewhat puzzled as to why I should find their workplace and its routines of such absorbing interest. They took the opportunity both formally (in the seminars and lectures I was asked to lead at the hospital), and informally (over meals or on the ferry), to exchange ideas about mental health issues.

One of the more unusual aspects of the research for me was that the meaning of confidentiality was very different. Divulging any information which might be interpreted as being of an official nature was fraught with difficulty. This was not a quirk of the hospital leaders but reflects a widely held world view in China. The concern with secrecy is embodied in the 1984 Statistics Law which requires that statistics be published regularly, but forbids the release of any data until political approval has been given. It also provides for the punishment of those in positions of leadership who make statistics public without prior approval. The policy that every datum is a state secret has stopped or greatly delayed the publication of most statistics (Banister, 1988).

Thus while the hospital officials were very co-operative in providing information about and access to patients, they were much more circumspect about the running of the hospital or matters concerning staff. This is not intended as a criticism. Within their world such caution is a matter of self-preservation and must be respected. The consequences, however, are that there are gaps in the data, and that partial impressions must sometimes suffice where a more systematic approach would have been desirable. For instance, permission could not be obtained for us to read any written, official statements relating to policy or administration within the hospital.

The Municipal Hospital is run by the city level of the Department of Civil Affairs. It was built in 1973 and was originally designed for patients who were classified as 'three have-nots'. It seems to have been anticipated from the start that the hospital would accept long-stay patients and its initial intake was largely long-term patients with no financial resources from the Department of Public Health hospital situated in the same city. According to staff at the hospital, nowadays 'three have-nots' patients are more likely to be 'two have-nots', in that they frequently have a family and possibly even employment, but do not have the financial resources to be able to afford hospitalisation.

The staff say that the hospital is now very different from when it started. At that time it was known as the Number Two Care and Education Home and employed only one qualified doctor. The staff and patients built the hospital on the site of a brickfield, an experience of camaraderie that some of the original staff and patients remember with warmth. Eventually the institution was promoted to being the Number One Care and Education Home and finally, at the beginning of the 1980s, was designated a Mental Hospital for Treatment and Rehabilitation.

The information that is presented here is a record of one particular hospital, at one particular time. The issue of time is important. In 1988, China was at the height of its financial growth, following ten years of the 'open-door policy' permitting greater economic freedom. Deng Xiaoping's strategy of developing the coastal areas first in the hope that there would be a trickle-down effect that would benefit the poorer, interior provinces had led to rapid development. Many of the peasants had taken advantage of the new policies to establish rural industries, acknowledged to be one of the major engines powering China's economic growth. But as Deng Xiaoping has always acknowledged, if you open the window to the aspects of Western technology that you want, some flies are bound to enter at the same time.

One of those flies was inflation. Another was the increasing disparity between the earnings of professional and white collar workers in the traditional organisations on the one hand, and individual entrepreneurs and peasants who were able to take direct advantage of the new economic policies, on the other. People accustomed to the common fellowship of deprivation found others' sudden wealth, through opportunity, talent or hard work, very difficult to stomach. There was also bitter resentment against the government concerning the rapidly rising costs of basic necessities, particularly food. This was most evident in people whose incomes were essentially fixed, like the staff at the hospital. Such people were not in a position to avail themselves of new economic opportunities and at the same time had to pay the price for others' success. On a general and individual level this led to a widespread outbreak of 'red eye disease', as jealousy is called.

This was also a time when the power of the Party to intervene in the running of enterprises and in people's lives was deliberately curtailed. The effects of this in the hospital will be discussed in more detail later. It was quite noticeable that, in comparison with reports produced by foreign visitors even in the late 1970s, there were no political study groups for staff, nor poster displays with any political content.

Location and physical environment

The hospital was situated on a tributary of a river at the very edges of the municipal administrative boundary. Indeed, the border between the city and province was formed by one of the hospital's perimeter fences. Thus the setting was essentially rural. The nearest market town was about 35 minutes away by bicycle. The hospital was surrounded by paddy fields, worked by humans and water buffalo, and commercial fishponds. It was possible to reach the hospital by road from the nearest big city, but it took over an hour and was impossible without individual transport as no bus route went near the place. The location of the hospital may be considered very typical of the tradition of building psychiatric hospitals in isolated spots.

For those staff who enjoyed the privilege of living in hospital quarters in the city (awarded usually after many years of service), rather than in quarters at the hospital, the day started early. During our stay there, when for two weeks we lived in the city rather than at the hospital, it meant arising reluctantly at 6 am, a walk to the bus stop during which we would consume breakfast of freshly steamed bread or a pork dumpling bought en route and a fight onto a bus whose passengers endured conditions that left them feeling envious of the luxury enjoyed by sardines. We had to be on time to catch the ferry that left at 7.30 am and arrived at the hospital at 8.45 am. The senior management team of the hospital enjoyed the privilege of being able to sit away from the rest of the passengers on the outside of the boat at the front. Other passengers, at least 50% of whom were hospital employees, sat in the body of the boat along with chickens, other assorted livestock and baskets of vegetables. They whiled away the journey chatting, playing cards and knitting.

Staff were expected to be on the ward by 9 am or 15 minutes after the ferry's arrival, and since we survived this routine for two weeks it was not hard to understand that they felt they had endured quite a hard day before they even arrived at work. Indeed the scheduling of the ferry and the sacrosanct two-hour lunch break were the major factors structuring the working day, which consisted of two and three-quarter hours in the morning and two and a quarter hours in the afternoon. Yet staff would not be back in the city before 6 pm and might well not reach home for another hour. This exhausting travel schedule almost certainly affected their efficiency at work.

The contrast between the 'outside' and the 'inside' of the hospital was very marked. The most remarkable aspect of the outside was the proximity of a holiday camp which shares grounds with the hospital. There was no physical separation, such as a wall or fence, between the two. This particular enterprise had been embarked upon by the previous Superintendent. The hospital was rich in land, but little else. Originally, it had been negotiated as a joint venture with a Japanese businessman who had promised US$ 2 000 000, while the hospital would provide the land. He withdrew from the project but the hospital went ahead with it in a modified form.

The camp has not been as successful as they would like. The hospital authorities attribute this to the proximity of a mental hospital, poor quality facilities, and the presence elsewhere of a much bigger and better equipped holiday camp that attracts many people. Of the facilities available, it seemed to be the hostel accommodation that was most popular with holiday-makers. It is possible that with the very crowded living conditions in the local city, where privacy is a scarce commodity, couples were using these facilities for romantic interludes. Thus the sign at the landing stage, rather than having the name of the hospital, says 'Welcome to the holiday camp'. Holiday-makers and patients (those who have ground privileges and others being taken on escorted walks by nurses), were frequently within sight of each other. They seemed to cope with this by ignoring each other; occupying the same space but different worlds.

Much thought and attention had been paid to landscaping the hospital grounds. There were traditionally inspired water gardens with rocks and pagodas and a profusion of flowering shrubs, plants and mature trees. It was extremely pleasant to walk or sit in the shade in the grounds. This made the contrast with the buildings, particularly the wards and the staff residences (which are the original wards built in 1973), even starker. The seven wards, built on the villa system, were separately located around the hospital grounds. Many of them had been built in the last five years but showed very marked signs of wear and tear. That this was not an inevitable consequence of shoddy workmanship or inferior materials was demonstrated by the hospital's new administration block which, while not luxurious, was pleasant and adequately maintained; and by the buildings associated with the holiday camp, like the dance hall, some of which were really quite well-built and attractive. While accepting that the conditions for the patients were not good, one of the senior doctors pointed out that those staff living in the original wards were even worse off. They shared a standpipe outside the buildings and used the outside toilets – ramshackle huts built over the edges of the numerous fishponds that were dotted around the hospital grounds.

Few facilities for staff or patients were provided. There were two small general shops or stalls, selling soft drinks, snacks, soap and so on. There was a staff canteen to provide the three major meals each day. Complaints about the standard of food were perennial, and the cook had recently been sent away on a course to improve his cooking skills. Vegetable and fruit sellers would come each morning, baskets perched precariously on their bicycles, to peddle their wares outside the canteen. Most of them were local peasants selling their own produce freshly picked that morning.

The patients

At the time of my research at the hospital, there were 630 patients, or 98.4% occupancy – a high figure by Western standards and a situation likely to increase the sense of stress among the staff. The hospital is quite large by Chinese norms for psychiatric hospitals and its population is primarily long-stay – 615 of the patients had been there for more than one year. The ratio of men to women was approximately 2:1; of both sexes, about 15% were aged between 16 and 30 years, nearly 40% were 31–45, 27% were 45–60, and 18% were over 61 years old. In 1987, admissions greatly exceeded discharges/deaths (135 against 34). This reflected a change of policy that required hospitals to be more self-supporting. The easiest way for the Municipal Hospital to do this was by admitting patients who paid rather than those who came under their traditional responsibility, the 'three have-nots'. Because of the long stay and indigent nature of their existing 'three have-not' patients the hospital authorities were not able to discharge this group to make room for the more lucrative 'self-payers'. Instead, the hospital authorities built another ward, thus substantially increasing their patient capacity.

Despite the change in policy of admitting more self-pay patients, the hospital still had 406 patients who were classified as the 'three have-nots'. There were very few of its other main responsibility, the veterans (8 patients); 216 patients were self-pay, almost all of whom were supported by their work unit.

There were no efforts to provide different conditions for the self-pay patients. They were kept on the same wards, received the same food and were subject to the same regime as the 'three have-nots' group. Veterans were entitled to extra fruit and snacks at festival times. Those who had served for a long time, or who gave especially meritorious service, also received cash bonuses which the hospital put in a savings account for them.

The largest diagnostic category was schizophrenia (84.7%; 534 patients) and the next was learning disability (10.9%; 69 patients). Fourteen patients had a diagnosis of organic psychosis; three were diagnosed as manic-depressive; and ten had other psychiatric illnesses.

Separate institutions for adults with a learning disability are very rare in China. The Municipal Hospital is thus typical of Chinese psychiatric hospitals in having a predominance of patients with the diagnosis of schizophrenia.

The treatment of choice was Western psychotropic drugs (81.9%; 516 patients). In collecting information from the patients' files there were no instances where Chinese medicine was being prescribed to control a psychotic disorder. It was used as a sedative or to improve physical health by 60 patients. Ten patients had received acupuncture and 18 had received ECT. The number who did not receive medication is not known.

The staff

There were 167 medical and technical staff, and 144 other staff. In terms of quantity, if not quality, the hospital was not especially understaffed, with one doctor for every 22.5 patients and one nurse per 5 patients. The hospital conforms to the Ministry of Civil Affairs' national guideline that there should be a staff–patient ratio of 1:2. This includes all staff, not just the doctors and nurses.

Problems centre more around the question of training. It seems that by Chinese standards the doctors in this hospital have had adequate training, most of them at the lower level, and almost all in Western medicine. In informal discussion with the staff, there was a discernible opinion that Western training was better. As one of the doctors commented, those trained in Western medicine "were proper medical men". Sixteen of the doctors had spent three years in medical college; four had spent three years and eight had spent five years or more at university.

Ten of the 28 doctors had 'specialised' in psychiatry; five of these had 3–10 years of psychiatric experience, the other five had over ten years. In the context of this hospital specialisation means that they had taken a six-month course on psychiatry organised by the City Bureau of Public Health (chronic illness section), in conjunction with the Chinese Medical Society and the Association of Neurology and Psychiatry. Each relevant unit was given a quota and were able to send doctors on full pay leave; this was optional, not compulsory, and relied on the motivation of the individual doctors. Eighteen doctors in the hospital had elected not to take this course, and were described as having specialised in other subjects. This inevitably affected the way that psychiatry was conceptualised, leading to a biological and somatic emphasis in treatment.

The doctors were ranked in a hierarchy at the top of which was an Assistant Chief Medical Officer. There were 14 Senior Medical Officers, nine Medical Officers and four Medical Assistants. One of the Senior Medical Officers and one of the Medical Officers were trained in Chinese medicine.

It would be difficult to prove, but it seemed that some of the new doctors employed by the hospital had agreed to come and work there because it was the only way they could come back to their home city. It was common practice in the past, when there were fewer universities or tertiary training institutes, to send fresh graduates to the remoter provinces. Thus many medical graduates from the provincial capital were sent elsewhere.

Most Chinese people have a visceral attachment to their 'home place', and if they cannot live there feel that they are in exile, even if still in China. Added to that, the standard of living and facilities locally are much higher than in most other places. Once sent away it is difficult to arrange to come back. One newly arrived doctor had been a dermatologist in a hospital in an interior province for 20 years. Listening to her talk, it seemed evident that she had struck a deal by agreeing to work in a very unpopular speciality in return for being permitted to return home. It is unlikely that she was the only one to employ this strategy.

Nurses had very low levels of training. Only 21 out of 126 had trained in a formal institution. Others might have studied by themselves to take the provincial level exams, and there was a day release course. However, this involved working on a Sunday and in the evening, and was unsuitable for those who had to work shifts or who had children. This, of course, included many of the nurses.

Furthermore, these examinations were of general, not psychiatric, nursing. Trained nurses may have a reasonable level of competence in the physical aspects of nursing, but there is very little of that which is appropriate or common to a psychiatric setting.

There was one chief nurse, 11 senior nurses and 52 nurses. Nearly half of the nursing staff consisted of nursing assistants (of whom there were 62) who had no formal training at all and who had learned what they knew from watching others on the wards. The nurses freely admitted that the nursing assistants did the same kind of work as full nurses, and that there was very little effective difference in their jobs. Most of the nursing staff had 3–10 years' experience (53 staff), and 26 staff had over ten years.

Administration

Remuneration is clearly a matter of great concern in any organisation for both management and workers. General issues concerning the structure of take home pay, particularly the issue of bonuses, were outlined in Chapter 3. What follows is an example of how this works in practice.

The highest increment in any grade was the lowest point of the next grade. The annual increment in any grade was 50 fen extra per month so that the maximum increment for seniority was about 20 yuan after 40 years of service. The starting salaries for medical or nursing assistants were between 50 and 60 yuan per month; those for medical officers and registered nurses were between 70 and 80 yuan; senior medical officers and the chief nurse started on 117 yuan.

These salaries were far too low to live on. Consequently, take home wages included a significant amount of what were technically bonuses, which were many and various. It is traditional in Chinese societies for workers to receive the 'thirteenth month', which is an extra month's pay at the time of the Spring Festival. At the hospital, 66% of this was guaranteed but the other 33% depended on performance. Everyone received a bonus of 30 yuan a month, and another one that was based on the local cost of living, which also came to about 30 yuan a month. Working in the mental health field is considered 'high risk', so they received an extra one yuan per working day as danger money. They were paid a travelling allowance of 20 yuan per month and a fuel allowance of

10 yuan. The hospital authorities also tried to provide some benefits in kind for the staff like washing powder, soap, and soft drinks in the summer. Uniforms and shoes were provided and housing was subsidised. All staff, from the superintendent to the gardener, received the same bonuses.

To give an example, the Medical Superintendent's basic salary was 100 yuan a month. This was for two reasons. First, he was a medical officer, the most junior grade of qualified doctor. Second, there are three grades of medical superintendent in China and the position at the hospital was at the lowest level of the three superintendent grades. Including the additional month's salary spread over the year, he received 126 yuan per month in bonuses, which was over 60% of his take home pay. Status and authority within the Communist system are not necessarily related to wages. The Medical Superintendent was paid less than the senior medical officers or even the cook. But the cook was aware of who wielded the real power. As he said, "I may earn more, but the Medical Superintendent could have me transferred anywhere in China tomorrow if he wanted".

Management structure

Authority relations were rigid and hierarchical. There were few formal consultation channels with staff and little room for innovation or change unless introduced either from the management team or by outside forces, as when the hospital became responsible for raising some of its own funding. Thus the structure depends largely on the top–down imposition of policies. At the same time, it is not easy for the management to change the working habits and patterns of the staff who, presumably, are pursuing their own agendas, which are not necessarily the same as those of the hospital management.

There was no organisation chart available in the hospital, and information had to be pieced together. The five most important people in the hospital hierarchy were the Party Secretary, the Medical Superintendent, the Deputy Medical Superintendent, the Medical Director and the Administrative Director (who was also a doctor, and in 1989 was promoted to become Medical Superintendent). Contrary to Western expectations, the most important, powerful person in the hospital was the Party Secretary, which was the case in any organisation or enterprise. All professional and administrative matters were subject to Party dogma and discipline.

Just as the Party is paramount at the national level, it is also expected to be paramount within each unit, whether that is a government department, a factory or a village (Madsen, 1984). When the manager of a unit and the Party Secretary of that unit were in disagreement, the Party Secretary would prevail and he had a license to interfere in any aspect of the business of the unit. As a possible example within the context of the Municipal Hospital, if the Party Secretary thought that insufficient time was being devoted to the political education of the patients, he could order the doctors to change the treatment regime.

In the Municipal Hospital, the Party Secretary was a veteran who had spent 18 years in the army and seen active service in the border conflict between China and Vietnam in 1979. One of his most treasured possessions was a white enamel mug (from which he always drank his tea), that commemorated this event and had only been given to those who had fought.

His official job description, which he had hung on his office wall, read:

1. Under the leadership of seniors and the Party branch, constantly ensure that the policy and decisions made by the Party branch are carried out consistently. Also to understand and investigate into policies of the Party.
2. Act as leader to implement the Party's organisation and propaganda. Plan and organise political work and evaluate and assess it regularly.
3. Work hard at learning the business of your unit. Act as a leader to cultivate the Party's good traditions and ways of doing things.
4. Investigate and research thoroughly to obtain a complete understanding of the hospital staff's thoughts and work and to develop the political thoughts of the staff.
5. Work fully as a staff member of the unit and help the superintendent to perform his role. Actively help and support their work.
6. Do well in the personnel and security work. Also work with youth, workers and women.

The impression was that the Party Secretary did not exert undue influence on staff. There were no political study groups, and political study was not seen as relevant for patients. During an informal conversation, the hospital cook said that people no longer wished to become Party members, and that the numbers recruited in recent years had dropped dramatically.

The seventh plenary session of the Twelfth National Party Central Committee held in October 1987 adopted the policy that the functions of the Party and government at all levels be separated.

(*Beijing Review*, 12 December 1987, p. 14). Managerial and professional considerations were to take precedence in the selection of the enterprise leader. In the hospital in the summer of 1988, they were still grappling with what this meant for them. The Party Secretary said in one interview that the job description on his wall, a lengthy treatise on the need to carry out and instruct on the policies of the Party, no longer applied.

Yet he clearly thought about and talked about himself as the major power in the hospital. He said that if there was a conflict between administrative and professional matters it was still his responsibility to resolve it. His major areas covered discipline, security and administration. Although the Medical Superintendent was now supposed to be responsible for personnel, the Party Secretary spoke about delegating this to him, and about the Medical Superintendent coming to consult him before any decisions were made. He concluded that as far as he was concerned nothing much had changed.

Thus during the period in which the research was undertaken, the Party Secretary was technically subordinate to the Medical Superintendent. However, this may be seen as essentially an anomaly. Following the Tiananmen incidents in 1989, the structure reverted to its previous position.

There is also a Chief Nurse who has not been included as it was not possible to ascertain where she would fit in, or indeed precisely what her responsibilities were. She was never included in any discussions in which I took part, unlike the other five. This could have been for a number of reasons; perhaps because she was a woman, and was not accepted by a predominantly male group, or because nurses were considered to be of lower status (even though in her case she earned more than the Medical Superintendent). What is also unclear is how the responsibilities of the Chief Nurse overlapped with those of the Medical Director. He described himself as being responsible for all the doctors and nurses on the wards.

The Administrative Director's job was described as being one with responsibility for administrative work, drafting the rules and regulations, paperwork, and writing reports. As well as the deputy, there was an assistant to the deputy and clerical workers.

Financing the hospital

The Municipal Hospital produced no substantive policy statements, which have to be taken from national rather than local material.

The Statistical Report of the Civil Affairs Bureau, 1987 (*Sheshui Baozhang Bao,* March 1988, p. 3) stated that:

> "Under the leadership of the Party and the Government and with the assistance of various departments, the Civil Affairs Ministry at all levels has persisted in the principles of reformation and openness and also launched the campaign of increasing production and income through curbing expenditure. The Civil Affairs Ministry has contributed to the development of a national stable economy, national economic reform and a stable society."

Translated into local terms this refers to the alteration of policy regarding the 'three have-nots', and the change to accepting paying patients in order to become more financially self-sufficient and less of a drain on the public purse. It is also reflected in the introduction of the 'contract responsibility' system within the hospital.

Finance was a delicate matter and one about which it was not easy to ask direct questions. The new system of financial responsibility laid a heavy burden on the shoulders of the Medical Superintendent, who had exercised considerable ingenuity in using the natural resources of the hospital to produce income.

The hospital's funding came from two sources. First was a block grant from the municipal government. In 1988 this was 1.1 million yuan; it generally increased each year to take account of rises in the cost of living. Grants for any capital projects had to be requested separately. The element of the grant that covered salaries was based on the number of 'three have-nots' patients, of whom there were about 400. The official staff ratio is one staff to two patients, and they have 640 beds, so they have to raise the money for the other staff themselves. The grant also covers accommodation, meals and treatment costs for all patients but no extras. Renovations, repairs and environmental improvements cannot be financed from the grant. The total expenses of the hospital were 1.6 million yuan, so that left the hospital with 500 000 yuan to find each year.

They had various ways of doing this. Renting out the hospital's fishponds to commercial fish farmers brought in about 20 000 yuan; the out-patients department generated 20 000; rent from the holiday camp managers contributed another 100 000. Self-pay patients were charged about 200 yuan per month. The hospital was permitted to keep about 30% of the fee income and used it to fund staff bonuses. Among other things, bonuses were used to raise staff salaries to levels comparable with similar jobs in the local city. They were subject to a departmental audit each year.

Money from the block grant not spent in one financial year was carried over to the next year.

Obviously, these figures do not entirely tally. Income from non-patient sources totalled approximately 140 000 yuan per annum. There were 216 self-pay patients. Assuming they all paid 200 yuan a month that would give an annual fee income of 518 400 yuan, 30% of which the hospital could keep. This leaves a shortfall of over about 200 000 yuan. It seems safe to assume that this is not the complete picture. If the grant and the total expenditure are correct, which seems reasonably likely, then the hospital was responsible for raising approximately 30% of its yearly expenditure. It would be surprising if this did not loom large in the mind of the Medical Superintendent whose responsibility it was to find this money.

The out-patients department

The main purpose of the out-patients department was to service the ward areas with an X-ray unit, pathology department, sterilising unit, pharmacy and discharged patients' records. Its secondary purpose was to provide a clinic for surrounding villages, the nearest clinic being about 25 minutes away by bicycle. Out-patient consultation was 30 fen plus the cost of the medication, and 50 fen for a specialist consultation. The department had its own staff of 24 including a pharmacist and technicians.

The hospital authorities were well aware that setting up the clinic helped to improve relations with people in the surrounding countryside who might otherwise have resented having a psychiatric hospital in their midst. It provided a cheap, convenient, primary care service, 24 hours a day. About 30–40 people were seen each day.

Life on the wards

There were four male wards, two female wards and one mixed ward for patients suffering from infectious diseases. This latter was divided into male and female sides with the only possible connecting route being through the treatment room and doctors' office, which occupied a no man's land in the middle. In fact, most of the patients in this ward were not suffering from a current infectious illness but may have done so in the past. Many of them were over 50 years old.

Physical environment

The emphasis on security in the hospital was largely within the ward, not at the perimeter. All wards had only one exit to the outside which was constantly locked. The gate was made either from solid metal or metal bars. Each ward had a courtyard where, at least in summer, most patients seemed to spend much of the day. Rooms had either four, six or eight beds in them. Only the 'service group' (privileged patients who do domestic work) in each ward were allowed to keep any individual possessions. Some of them were provided with a locker while others kept a bag under their beds. The majority of patients did not have a sheet on the bed: that was a privilege reserved for members of the service group. The limited number of sheets available were obtained by the Superintendent, second-hand at bargain prices, from a hostel that was closing down. All the other patients had a rattan mat to cover the boards in an iron bedstead (a very common practice in China). Most beds seemed to have a mosquito net but there were no fans, a necessity rather than a luxury in a sub-tropical climate.

The wards, almost without exception, were completely bare of any decoration. There were no photographs, no calendars, no pictures cut from a magazine, no souvenirs of the patients' past life or individual identity at all. The only exception was that service group members sometimes had a potted plant by their beds, but that hardly provided any connection to a life outside the hospital. The doctors' room on each ward was slightly livelier, with the occasional calendar, picture, vase of flowers or potted plant. So the concept of enlivening the environment did exist.

Each ward had one large room with tables and chairs, which doubled as a place to sit and a dining room, although not every ward had space for all patients to sit at the same time. Many took their meals standing or squatting in the courtyard. Most courtyards had no benches or seats – they had no choice but to sit or squat on the ground.

There was one exception to the general air of bleakness – male Ward L's garden. This was quite clearly the pride and joy of a dedicated group of green-fingered enthusiasts among both the staff and patients of the ward, and was magnificent. Patients were able to sit out in it and receive visitors there. The staff said quite plainly that as patients had contributed to it, they should also be allowed to enjoy it. Another male ward had a roof garden mostly consisting of potted plants. However, it had no wall or guard at the edge so only service group members were able to use it, under supervision.

Even by standards of mainland China, the toilet and bathing facilities were basic. The toilets were concrete channels in the floor with the cubicles separated by half walls, and had no doors. This is not so unusual, but there were never more than six toilets for between 90 to 100 patients, and some of those were not accessible during the day. Bathing facilities varied slightly but normally consisted of cold water taps set about three feet up the wall opposite the toilet cubicles. There was absolutely no privacy at all and the design clearly facilitated being able to wash a group of patients at the same time. Another version involved a bath large enough to hold seven people at once, with a large rubber hose lying inside, presumably to hose them down.

Ward staffing structure

There were 24 staff on each ward. There were always three doctors (one of whom was in charge), a head nurse, two workmen, and a general duties nurse. The balance in each ward was then split between nurses and nursing assistants, with the latter always outnumbering the former. No significant difference could be detected between the wards in the distribution of nurses although there were minor variations. The general duties nurse covered tasks like keeping a record of patients' allowances, administering special food rations and other benefits for veterans, and controlling and dispensing toilet paper, soap, sanitary towels and so on. She was sometimes called the 'odd job nurse'. Patients wanting to use toilet paper, soap and so on had to request it from the nursing staff.

Nursing regimen

It is a national policy in Ministry of Civil Affairs psychiatric hospitals that patients are divided into four nursing categories (Zhang Dejiang, 1986; Sun *et al*, 1987). It may also be true of the hospitals in the Ministry of Public Health system (Tousley, 1985).This policy was implemented at the Municipal Hospital and the four levels are outlined below:

Level 0 – refers to patients who require complete bed rest and intensive nursing care. These patients are generally elderly.

Level 1 – all newly admitted patients or patients who are relapsing are allocated to this level, as well as any others who are considered to have a serious psychiatric problem. These patients are generally carefully watched and supervised by nursing staff.

Level 2 – the illness of patients at this level is considered to be under control, and the condition of the patient steadily improving. At this level patients may be expected to look after their own daily needs and basic hygiene with little supervision.

Level 3 – the Ministry of Civil Affairs' encyclopaedia (Sun *et al,* 1987) defines these patients as having "their mental illness syndrome basically removed", and being ready to be discharged. In the context of the Municipal Hospital, where discharge is a rare option, these are patients who can go out without supervision and are generally independent. They are also in the service groups (see below).

All staff were very aware of the necessity of maintaining the 'three preventions', that is to prevent suicide, prevent hurt to others and prevent running away. Patients who were considered to be in danger of any of these three actions were dubbed 'three prevention' patients and would become the subject of very careful supervision. If a patient in this category did manage to commit any of the three actions, the staff would be subject to severe criticism. If a patient not in this category committed any of these acts, the staff would also be severely criticised for making a wrong assessment of the patients' mental state. Tousley makes similar observations, and comments on how stressful psychiatric nurses in China find the responsibility of preventing suicide (Tousley, 1985).

Patients' files

Standardised ward files were kept on all patients. Information included a record of nursing care, long and short-term prescriptions, reports of accessory investigations and tests, a case record since hospitalisation began, a record of mental condition, and temperature and blood pressure charts. It was a requirement that each patient must have a comment recorded on his or her file by one of the ward doctors each month, although some of these comments were perfunctory in the extreme.

The hospital had been making a great effort to improve the quality and organisation of the information on its patients' files. While we were there, a lengthy series of meetings was in progress to try to decide on the changes. One that had been agreed was the need to include much more information about the patients' family and social background, although even the newer files that I read showed little evidence that the policy had been implemented. There was also concern about the way that diagnoses were being reached. One of the new rules was that doctors should diagnose through exclusion.

Daily schedule and activities

There is a nationally stated policy about the regime in psychiatric hospitals run by the Ministry of Civil Affairs:

> "The mental hospital run by the Ministry of Civil Affairs is using an integrative therapeutic treatment for the patients. This therapy includes medical treatment, work treatment, recreational treatment, and psycho-ideological treatment. These four treatments, integrated together, form the 'four integration treatment'. The medical treatment controls the relapse of mental patients, the work treatment trains the patients to adapt to social functions, the recreational treatment helps the patients to build up their physique, and education trains the patients to recover from mental disabilities and to improve their mental health." (Sun *et al*, 1987)

While the 'four integrations' was practised in the Municipal Hospital, staff repeatedly said that it involved concentrating on drugs, occupation, recreation and physical exercise. They did not mention ideological treatment. They did sometimes say that it was important to educate patients about the facts of mental illness, but there was never any implication that there were political overtones to this. When specifically asked whether they thought that political education had any place to play in the treatment of mental illness, the doctors were very clear that it was of little or no use. It seems that, knowingly or not, the staff at the hospital have reshaped the 'four integrations' to be more to their taste.

Patients were woken up at about 6 am and washing and toileting took place. Breakfast was at 7 am followed by medications. Patients were supposed to make their own beds and keep their rooms tidy. The morning staff meeting took place at 9 am, when patients who did not have a peaceful night were discussed, physical ailments reported on, and duties allocated for the day. Sometimes the doctor in charge used this opportunity to issue a general instruction, like reminding staff to make sure that patients were warm enough at night, or to keep a special eye on those patients who were sad because they have no relatives to go to during festival times. (The major festivals are the Spring Festival, which usually falls in February, marking the beginning of the new year according to the lunar calendar, and the Mid-Autumn, or Moon, Festival.)

After this meeting, all patients, and technically all staff, were supposed to spend 15 minutes engaged in physical exercises led by one of the staff. Participation seemed largely perfunctory on the part of both staff and patients. Patients were then mostly locked out of their rooms so that they could not go back to bed, and most frequently locked into the courtyard. Some were called to the treatment room to have their blood pressure taken, escorted for an X-ray, or had small injuries attended to. This was also the time when hair and nail cutting took place. Some nurses went round tidying patients' beds and rooms. About twice a week, those patients who were able were taken for a walk by the nurses. The destination was often the grounds of the holiday camp, but in fact most of the facilities there (like the swimming pool, or the small 'dodgems') were not in working order. There was an open air pool table which patients sometimes used. There were other facilities, such as a dance hall, but those did not seem to be used by patients. The hospital had its own activities hall.

Lunch was at 11 am, followed by medications. From about 12.30 pm to 2.30 pm patients were allowed back into their rooms to take a nap. There appeared to be very little activity on the wards during the afternoon. There was more medication at 3.30 pm and again at 8.15 pm; the final meal of the day was at 5 pm and bed time was at 10 pm.

There was no occupational therapy department or activity centre at the hospital. Nothing in the way of normal recreational activities (knitting, reading, painting, calligraphy) was provided on a daily, routine basis to keep patients' brains active and functional. Thus for most patients the ward was their entire world. In such circumstances, the quality of both the relationships with staff and the ward regime assume particular importance. The major occupational activity provided on the ward was pulling pieces of cotton apart in order that it could be rewoven. This was piece work and patients were paid a small amount for what they did. It was mind-numbingly boring work, although staff claimed that patients were not capable of anything more complicated. On some wards, patients engaged in this activity were permitted to watch television at the same time to relieve the boredom.

One ward (M) was exceptional in this respect in that staff had arranged for another money-earning activity for patients: sticking labels on packets. Staff had also spent bonus money that they had earned helping to whitewash hospital buildings to buy a table tennis table and equipment, and a badminton net and racquets for patients. Both activities took place in the courtyard. Ward M was also the only ward where both staff and patients smoked openly.

Each ward had a colour television and the hospital had a video player (a sign of the level of affluence in this area), so films were also occasionally shown. There appeared to be no newspapers for patients on any of the wards, although a newspaper is an essential part of life for many Chinese people under ordinary circumstances. Only on one ward was a single boardgame observed, Chinese chequers, and staff were never seen interacting with individual or small groups of patients on the ward in a 'recreational' way, other than occasionally leading group singing.

While the lack of any meaningful daily occupation was one of the most obvious comments to be made about the daily schedule, the Medical Superintendent put a slightly different light on the matter. He said that the previous Superintendent, under whom he had worked, insisted that all patients should do four hours daily labour, unless thcy were so ill or aged as to make it impossible. He felt this was an unreasonable demand given the type of patients for whom they catered, and stopping the practice was one of the first things he had done on becoming Superintendent.

There was little effort made to orient patients towards the outside world, unless it was through watching television. They had no reminders of their own past life; no photographs of any sort, no souvenirs, no treasured objects. Nor were they encouraged to take any interest in what might be going on in the outside world. Obviously money was limited but opportunities that would cost nothing were ignored, for instance, by using televised national or international events, such as the Olympics, that involved China.

Most wards told us that they had recently started organising trips to the city once or twice a year (the zoo or the sports stadium were the two places most frequently mentioned), and that they tried to take as many patients on these trips as they possibly could. Such outings were very popular with the patients – the staff reported that they opened up more as a consequence.

Visitors were encouraged to come at any time during office hours (9 am to 4 pm) on any day of the year, although nurses preferred them to arrive after 9.30 am, when the handover was finished. They did not have to give notification of their visit. The staff wished more relatives would visit the hospital, as nothing made the patients unhappier than the sense that they had been abandoned by their families. Very few made the effort. Visiting was difficult because of the remoteness of the hospital.

The ward environment was grossly understimulating. For the majority of patients, there was almost nothing to do, day in and day out. There was no provision for the encouragment of individual talents, and no group activities or games, except on special occasions. There were no inter-ward table tennis contests, no Friday night socials.

Psychiatric hospitals in the UK used to be criticised for providing for all the needs of the patients under one roof, obviating the necessity for them ever to go out. But this hospital provided for little other than patients' physical needs; nor were they able to go out. While the hospital authorities were limited in what they could do to promote discharge for many of the patients, there were many ways in which the regime could have been humanised and conditions for patients improved.

The service groups

Each ward had about ten patients in a service group. They were under the immediate direction of the two domestic workers, and their basic duties were to help with the cleaning, and to assist in looking after the more incapable patients. Their cleaning duties were called the 'Three Front Door Responsibilities'. These amounted to keeping the ward clean, and attempting to improve the environment. In return they were paid a small allowance of 3–5 yuan a month; they could also keep some personal possessions, bath when they wished, go for walks unescorted, and have a sheet on their bed. Only one patient appeared ever to wear her own clothes occasionally. One ward permitted patients to have their own underwear as long as they took responsibility for washing it. Most patients had no underwear and were dressed in hospital pyjamas.

Admission and discharge procedures

The official way for a patient to be referred to the hospital was through the work unit or family. Whoever made the referral contacted the hospital. The hospital sent a doctor from whichever ward had an empty bed to assess the patient at his home or work place. If the doctor thought he was suitable for admission he recommended this to the Superintendent, Deputy or Medical Department head. Relatives, work unit colleagues, or occasionally the police would then bring the patient to the hospital.

This was the theory but it was clear from reading the files that many patients were brought to the hospital to be seen for the first time, and were then admitted straight away. A number of the patients were tricked by relatives into thinking that they were going on a picnic, or being taken somewhere for a job interview. As one head doctor commented, "many patients arrive handcuffed and think they are coming to a prison. They wonder 'what have I done wrong? Have I been anti-revolutionary?'".

While we were travelling to the hospital on the ferry one morning, we overheard a conversation between the ferry captain and the Medical Superintendent. The captain had a 15-year-old relative who was hearing voices and who had attempted suicide, and he wanted to know how he could have her admitted to the hospital. The Department of Public Health hospital had already refused to admit her, although no reason was given. The Medical Superintendent's answer was simple. A deposit of 500 yuan was needed and a document from the girl's work unit, or that of her parents, or her neighbourhood organisation, saying that they would take her back and be responsible for the fees. He appeared to be willing to admit the girl without ever having seen her.

Discharge seemed to depend on a number of factors. The most important was whether or not the patient had a work unit or family willing to accept responsibility. The lack of either made the chances of discharge extremely remote, whatever the condition of the patient. There may have been some liaison between the ward doctors and the relatives or work unit. One doctor described discharging a patient home without any warning to the relatives, so that they had no opportunity to refuse to accept her. The doctor simply escorted the patient back to the city, took her to the family home and left her there. There is no evidence to suggest that this is a common occurrence.

Some wards maintained contact with patients after they had been discharged. Doctors in one ward claimed that they visited discharged patients once a month. Those on another ward said they paid them a visit once or twice a year. This did not form part of their official work and they did it out of kindness. They said that no fee was charged.

Home leave

A surprisingly large number of patients was permitted to go on home leave, particularly at festival times. In female Ward P, 40 patients went home. Other wards routinely permitted ten or so patients to go home on leave. Some travelled independently, while others were escorted by their relatives. Staff were aware that there were a number of patients who were quite well enough to live outside, but whose families were not prepared to have them on anything other than a temporary basis. Some patients were unwilling to be discharged because they felt that they were a burden on their families. One woman, who was described as 'very capable', used to go home at harvest time to help her family. But one year her brother died while she was there, and the next year her nephew drowned, and she now refuses to go home, although her family are quite willing to take her, because she feels she brings disaster on their heads.

Extended leave was also used inventively, as follows:

(a) To send patients back to their work units, so that if they relapsed there was a guarantee that the hospital would take them back again.

(b) To encourage patients to keep taking medication because they knew they could be recalled instantly.

(c) To persuade a work unit to accept someone from the hospital (who was not originally their employee), give them a job, and house them. In these circumstances the patient was on extended leave because of the advantages outlined above, and because the work unit was then absolved from paying the fee if the patient relapsed.

The use of seclusion

Each ward had at least two, and sometimes as many as six, seclusion rooms. On the more modern wards, each seclusion room was entirely enclosed and soundproofed. The rooms were not padded, and generally were furnished with only a bed or sometimes a mat on the concrete floor. The doors were made from metal, and there was a small grille high up in the door that permitted staff to look in. In the older wards the design was somewhat different. On female Ward P the seclusion rooms were by the main door. To enter them one went through a locked, barred metal door into a short corridor, on either side of which, facing each other, were three cells. Each was locked and had a barred metal door, so that occupants were visible to each other all the time.

The impression gained was that staff were not entirely at ease in talking about these rooms, or the uses to which they were put. On one ward we were told that they had not been used for over a year – but then, at the handover, part of the discussion centred on the behaviour of a patient who had been in the seclusion room for some days. Some wards said they now only used them for patients who were physically ill; others that they were used for patients who were relapsing or misbehaved, but "only for a few days".

From what we were told and what we could observe, there were grounds for concern. There were no hospital guidelines for the use of seclusion, thus decisions about who went in them, and the duration of their stay, remained at the whim of individual members of staff or shifts. Nor did there seem to be any requirement to inform the Medical Director if a seclusion room was being used.

In female Ward P we were told of a patient who had been kept in seclusion for ten years because she bit other patients occasionally. She had only been released about four months previously and had apparently not bitten anyone since then. One of the doctors who had been there for ten years described the previous head ward doctor as very conservative, with only basic medical training, although she had worked in psychiatry for 30 years. It was she who had locked the patient up. The implication was that the regime had improved under the new head ward doctor.

Another instance was given on male Ward M of a patient who had been placed in a seclusion room for 20 years because he was "a severe sexual pervert". His offences seemed to be masturbation, some form of sexual assault (but not rape), and writing political graffiti on the walls about national leaders. He had recently been released, and staff said that they successfully control his behaviour through medication and the judicious granting or withholding of cigarettes and favourite food.

The Deputy Medical Superintendent told us that there were rules to forbid staff hitting or shouting at patients, and that the expectation was that staff would be able to control patients' behaviour within three days through medication. This should have obviated the extended use of seclusion but the indications were that it did not.

Staff discipline

According to the Medical Director, there was a code of practice for the whole hospital, and his concern was to encourage people to work according to these standards, rather than to punish them when they did not. He felt that some people criticised him for this view. Discipline tended to be enforced by manipulating the bonus element in wages, and by holding the entire staff of a ward or the whole shift responsible for mistakes committed by one person. If he considered that the head nurse and doctor of a ward had sincerely tried to rectify mistakes made by themselves or their staff, then the Medical Director would not penalise all the staff by reducing their bonus. It seemed that if a member of staff made minor errors, the ward might decide to reduce that person's bonus, awarding an equivalent amount to another staff member who had performed exceptionally well.

Evaluation was supposed to be carried out daily by the head doctor and nurse at the handover in the morning. Sometimes mistakes were pointed out publicly to increase the alertness of other staff (see also Henderson & Cohen, 1984). Sometimes it was done individually. There was also evaluation from the Medical Department whose members went to each ward to give supervision. Sometimes ward senior staff, but not the head doctor or nurse, reported mistakes direct to the Medical Department. Views varied as to whether the Medical Department should deal with this directly, or refer it to the ward's head doctor. On the wall of the doctor's office in each ward was a 'mistakes chart', with the name of every staff member of that ward on it. Mistakes were publicly recorded and graded according to four levels of severity. There was also a 'mistakes book' on each ward and this was used at the end of each month to calculate the bonus for all staff members.

How this worked in practice was demonstrated by the procedures invoked when patients ran away. The ward reported the disappearance to the hospital office. It was the duty of the staff on the ward at that time to search for the patient. If they could not find the patient the matter was reported to the public security bureau. According to new rules laid down by the Medical Department, all staff on that shift had to take the blame, whether they were directly involved or not, and all would have their bonuses reduced. Penalties were higher if the patient came to any harm, or caused any harm, while out of the hospital. In that case a 'big, black mark' would be recorded on each staff person's file. Three of these administrative marks were supposed to lead to instant dismissal. No one had ever been dismissed from the hospital, and one wonders how effective these deterrents were. It is difficult to persuade people to undertake this kind of work and the Medical Director must have been aware of this when disciplining staff. Perhaps that is why he tried to rely on persuasion rather than punishment.

On the evidence available from talking to staff, reading files, and ward observation, it seems unlikely that the supervision techniques described by the Medical Director are effective in raising and maintaining standards of care. While the upper echelons of the hospital medical hierarchy may have had a clear idea of what proper practice in the hospital should be, there seemed to be major problems in operationalising that throughout the hospital. The impression gained was that ward doctors were resistant to what they saw as interference. Nor did the head ward doctors seem to take much lead in monitoring professional standards in their wards, for instance, by checking through files or ensuring that proper diagnoses were carried out. Good standards seemed to rely more on individual interest and diligence, which occurred in small pockets around the hospital, rather than being an agreed common goal.

140   *Mental Health Care in China*

The contract system on the wards

Since its introduction, the 'contract responsibility system' has tended to permeate every aspect of life in China. Within the hospital it was used in diverse ways, from a basis for hiring staff to rationing soap. The idea behind it is to break the 'iron rice bowl' (a guaranteed job for life, independent of ability or motivation), and to force people to accept responsibility for their own actions, by setting quotas and making at least part of their salaries reflect their work achievement.

Within the hospital, the contract responsibility system was used in a number of ways. Various kinds of staff were employed on a contract basis, including a few of the doctors. Mostly these terms were offered to nurses, maintenance staff, the carpenter and the cook, although it was still more common for staff to be permanent and therefore allocated to the job. The basic salary for contract staff varies in different areas of China according to living standards, and from enterprise to enterprise according to the material wealth and workload of the unit. The contract is usually for two or three years and there is a probationary period of one year, after which the salary is increased. Once a contract is finished it may be renewed, usually at a higher salary. Contracts give more flexibility to both staff and management over choice of job, wage levels and personnel. But they may also make people feel very insecure, particularly those used to the 'iron rice bowl'.

Although the hospital had never dismissed a member of staff, there had been times when a contract had not been renewed. If a contract was not renewed the government provided a proportion of the original salary (but not including the bonuses), for 6 to 12 months to cushion the search for new employment. Both employees and the work unit paid into a contributory pension scheme for contract workers, which might be paid as a gratuity at the end of a contract if the person left, or as an old age pension on retirement.

Other areas of the hospital were also affected by the use of contracts. The workload of patients' laundry was contracted out to existing staff and their families. Security was semi-contracted out. Those working in that section were originally staff members, but as a way of increasing their performance they were paid a bonus at the end of the year if there had been no cases of theft or untoward incidents. Equally, they were financially penalised if there had been.

The out-patients department used to claim that it was too busy to perform routine urine, blood and stool examinations on in-patients. The hospital authorities therefore set up a target for them to fulfil, with the usual rewards and penalties operating through the bonus system. It took two to three months to establish workload statistics, and to persuade out-patients department staff to participate in the system. The Medical Director said that, while it was possible for the system to be abused by staff performing unnecessary tests, this did not happen very often and if they noticed it going on, they talked to the staff, and in extreme circumstances deducted money from their bonuses.

At the time of our visit, the hospital authorities intended to introduce the contract system on the wards as a way to make staff aware of the resources that they were using, and to ensure that they were not wasteful. This would affect the use of electricity, patients' clothes, soap, toilet paper and so on. The Medical Director did not think that this would lead to goods being unnecessarily restricted in order that staff could increase their bonuses by remaining below the target. On the other hand, there does seem to be space for abuse in such a system, particularly since patients are not likely to be able to make effective complaints if their rations of toilet paper and soap become too sparse.

Differences between individual wards

Groups of staff were subjectively certain that the administration favoured some wards over others. The staff of male Ward N were quite sure that the Medical Director's department sent them the patients who were the hardest to manage. Information from the data collection forms was analysed by ward but no reliable statistical differences were found, although efforts in this direction were hampered by the small number of cases in each ward. Some wards did have more self-pay than 'three have-not' patients, and this may have made some difference.

The collective view of the staff was that the self-pay patients, being more acute, were more interesting and rewarding to treat. They also thought that standards in the hospital had risen since these patients were admitted, with more and better qualified doctors being employed. It is interesting to note that, while these patients may be considered to be more acute, this is not reflected in the discharge figures which have remained more or less the same for the last six years. This would suggest that self-pay patients are needlessly being turned into long-stay patients, because they are reliable sources of income, because the staff find them more rewarding and are reluctant to let them go, or because relatives are reluctant to take them back.

Male Ward N staff reported that their ward had deteriorated over the years. During the late 1970s, this was a rehabilitation ward with younger patients. Many of the patients worked in the grounds, and staff and patients played ball games together. Perhaps most significantly, the ward doors were open all day; now, as with all the other wards, they are permanently locked. As the patients have become older, they are not so lively, and the situation on the ward has deteriorated. This assessment is supported by the leaden ward atmosphere, and by the much heavier doses of drugs given to the patients on this ward than on others.

In contrast, male Ward M, while having similar physical conditions to male Ward N, gives a very different impression. The staff here seemed to be the rebels of the hospital, for instance both staff and patients smoked quite openly. The ward office contained various charts of information to do with their patients, such as the numbers of 'three have-nots' and self-pay, types of diagnoses, and the numbers taking drugs. They were proud of the fact that their patients earned the most money from pulling cotton threads, and it was this ward that had found another income source for patients, sticking labels on packets.

The staff were quite convinced that providing patients with occupation during the day prevented, or at least slowed down, deterioration and thought that the emphasis that they placed on this accounted for the better condition of their patients. This was in spite of the fact that over 90% of their patients were 'three have-nots', generally considered to be the least rewarding. This was also the ward where the staff spent some of their bonuses on providing extra facilities for patients. Whether or not their perceptions were objectively correct, they seemed to improve the staff 'spirit', and produce a sense of camaraderie lacking on other wards.

In some ways, it was easier to grasp the differences between the female wards because there were only two. Female Ward P was a livelier place to be. All staff working on both female wards knew that Ward P had the 'better' patients. Female patients being readmitted routinely requested to go to Ward P. Patients there would crowd around visitors asking questions and showing great interest in anything new or different. The hospital put only female staff on this ward, unlike female Ward Q which had all male doctors, because it was felt that the sexual temptation for male staff working with younger and livelier patients would be greater. Female Ward Q had older patients, and they certainly appeared less well-oriented than those on Ward P, although there was no way of knowing whether this was a result of longer hospitalisation, different ward regimes or the process of illness.

During discussion on the wards, all staff groups were asked in what ways they thought the hospital had changed over the years.

The most common replies were improvements in the physical setting, in standards of staffing and quality of staff, and thus improvements in treatment and maintenance of files. There had been two medical superintendents before the present one. Both of them had been retired army veterans with no experience of hospitals or medical background. Some staff spoke quite openly of the conditions in the past, when both physical and mental illnesses went untreated, and patients were left to die with little intervention. Thus, whatever the conditions seem like to an outsider, the staff, using a different but no less relevant frame of reference, have a more positive sense of the hospital.

Conclusions

As an institution, from the patients' point of view, the Municipal Hospital is a world enclosed upon itself in a way that would be near impossible to find in a UK hospital. Goffman's analysis of total institutions (1961) has been part of the professional air we breathe for so long that it comes as a shock to find a place seemingly innocent of all notions about the iatrogenic effects of institutions and unaware that patients' behaviour is a product of environment as well as of the disease process. His analysis is still relevant to the Municipal Hospital.

The hospital was physically isolated, which reinforced the institutional ethos of the place and severely reduced the opportunities for community-based treatment and rehabilitation. The staff who lived in the city, while seeing themselves as fortunate, paid a high price in the tiring journey that had to be made twice a day. If it was ever intended that the holiday camp would overcome the problems of isolation, it had not worked.

The hospital seemed in danger of creating new long-stay patients unnecessarily. If acute patients are to be admitted to what has been essentially a hospital for chronic patients, then thought should be given to how they are to be appropriately handled. Staff obviously thought that accepting acute patients had brought benefits to the hospital. Little thought seemed to have been given to what might be in the best interests of the patients.

The lack of trained staff and training facilities had a damaging effect on standards of patient care. This was particularly true of the nurses, who were allocated to nursing, psychiatric nursing and this hospital. Choice and voluntary adherence to a professional ethos had absolutely no part to play. Under such circumstances, exhortations by the Party 'to serve patients with all your heart' were utterly ineffectual. Attempts to manipulate the bonus system to produce better levels of patient care did not appear to work because the amounts of money involved were too small. It was also difficult to do anything more than discipline staff in a token way.

Basic physical needs were met as far as clothing, feeding and hygiene were concerned. The number of deaths each year, if accurately recorded, did not seem excessive. There also seemed to be an adequate, if basic, range and supply of psychotropic medication.

There was little attempt at ward management regarding the social, psychological and rehabilitation needs of patients. No varying regimes for different groups of patients had been implemented. It would have been possible to do this for those with an acute or chronic mental illness, as well as those patients with a learning disability. All wards had a number of patients with a learning disability. As a general rule, such people tend to respond better to a structured routine which usually features opportunities for education concerning the skills of daily living. For this to be implemented in the hospital, such an environment would need to be created on one specific ward.

There may have been management reasons for keeping the more able patients scattered around different wards in order that they could help with cleaning and caring for less able patients. However, it would seem fairer for them if they could live in a more open and independent environment, even if they were still in the hospital.

If the environment for the patients was an essentially punitive one, this was also true for staff. At least two issues raised their anxiety level. First, they believed that a significant number of patients were potentially violent and that they were working with dangerous people. Second, rather than being rewarded for good work, they were punished for mistakes. They lived with the spectre of 'what would happen if...?', even if their worst imaginings were rarely fulfilled. Such an atmosphere is not conducive to initiative or innovation. Instead, it encourages a 'head down' stance where sticking to the rule book is a means of protection.

Psychiatric care in China is not at a stage where it is able to identify the above issues as problems, and the standards of care in psychiatric hospitals have not yet been identified as a source of concern. The country (understandably) has other priorities. There are no complaints procedures, no independent inspection mechanisms; there is little communication between levels in the hierarchies, and no sense that hospitals need to be radically rethought. The lack of such mechanisms and procedures does not bode well for the patients.

6   The patients

An aim of this book is to build up as accurate picture as possible of the patients in the Municipal Hospital. They are not necessarily typical of all patients in psychiatric hospitals in China, but as our current level of knowledge about people in this position very low, even circumscribed understanding of a reliable nature is valuable. Two broad approaches were selected. The quantifiable information available in patients' files that gives an aggregate picture of who they are is presented in this chapter. In the following chapter various methodologies are used to reflect on the meaning that patients bring to their life experiences.

The information in this chapter is based on a data set of patients in the Municipal Hospital aged 16–60, with a firm diagnosis of schizophrenia. The decision to concentrate on schizophrenia was taken because over 80% of the patients have that diagnosis; also, there has been much controversy over the diagnosis of depression and neurasthenia in China (Kleinman, 1986; Young & Xiao, 1993).

Four hundred and sixty people fitted the criteria in terms of age-range and diagnosis and from them a random sample of 147 was drawn. The information was collected during September and October, 1988. Statistical analyses were performed using SPSS–PC.

Diagnosis

Do Chinese and Western doctors mean the same thing when they diagnose schizophrenia? The World Health Organization has been involved in a more or less continuous epidemiological research effort since 1966 to establish whether schizophrenia is a world-wide phenomenon. (World Health Organization, 1973, 1979; Sartorius *et al*, 1986).

Among what Jablensky (1988) calls their first rank findings is that the syndrome of schizophrenia is universal. Although no single symptom was invariably present in every patient and in each setting, the overall clinical configuration of the disorder was remarkably constant across cultures. Also, the subjective experiences of individuals suffering from schizophrenia and the way that they describe it are similar in people of very different backgrounds and educational experience (Jablensky, 1988).

The People's Republic of China did not take part in the WHO study, although Taiwan did; but the Chinese authorities have been concerned to carry out their own epidemiological survey, and to work on defining its own diagnostic criteria. In 1989 the Chinese Association for Neurology and Psychiatry met in Xian and accepted the report of a working party that became the *Chinese Classification and Diagnostic Criteria of Mental Disorders* (second edition), or CCDM–2. This is the fifth time since 1958 that the psychiatric diagnostic system has been revised but CCDM–2 (sometimes known as the 'Yellow Mountain' criteria) is more scientifically based and has been tested more extensively than the others. Consequently, it is likely to have more staying power.

Schizophrenia is defined in CCDM–2 as a group of mental illnesses with unknown cause. Onset is mostly in adolescence and young adulthood and is associated with disorders of sensation, thinking, affect behaviour and a lack of co-ordination in mental activities. In general, there is no disorder of consciousness or impairment of intelligence. The course of the illness is usually long.

The classification of schizophrenia in CCDM–2 seems to contain elements of ICD–9, ICD–10 and DSM–III–R. The Chinese classification recognises many forms of schizophrenia: hebephrenic, catatonic, paranoid and residual, all in both ICD–9 and DSM–III–R; undifferentiated (DSM–III–R); simple (ICD–9); atypical schizophrenia, which is divided into two parts – schizophreniform psychosis, which is not recognised as a form of schizophrenia by either international classification system, and post-schizophrenic depression (ICD–10); and 'other types' of schizophrenia which is not a classification recognised by either ICD–9 or DSM–III–R.

CCDM–2 specifies that before a firm diagnosis can be made, at least two of the following symptoms should be present. If the existence of a symptom is unclear or not typical then three symptoms are needed: disorder in thinking; auditory hallucinations; disordered behaviour (catatonia or foolish, child-like actions); the patient's belief that they are being controlled by others; thought broadcasting; thought blocking; disturbance of affect (apathy, giggling to self). CCDM–2 also requires that doctors diagnose by exclusion.

The major difference between CCDM–2 and DSM–III–R seems to be that the former permits a firm diagnosis to be made after three months from onset, while DSM–III–R requires six months. This probably reflects different attitudes towards labelling, with Western doctors reluctant to confirm a diagnosis that produces stigma and social handicap. These scruples are certainly no less in China but doctors say that they would be thought incompetent by relatives if they took six months to diagnose a disease! From my observations of practice, they rarely wait even three months.

There can be no doubt that schizophrenia exists in China and would be identified as approximately the same set of symptoms as recognised elsewhere. A trickier question remains to be answered. How many psychiatric doctors in China use CCDM–2? It is well documented in China that the tendency is to over-diagnose schizophrenia and under-diagnose depression and manic depression (Liu, 1980, 1983; Yan *et al*, 1982; Chen *et al*, 1984; Yan & Xiang, 1984; Yuan & Peng, 1987; Altschuler *et al*, 1988; Cheung, 1991). My own observations when reading files in several hospitals tend to confirm this. But, as Leff says with regard to the difficulty of persuading American doctors to change their diagnosing habits from their previous all-inclusive psychodynamic approach to the much stricter phenomenological guidelines of DSM–III–R, "official policy is one thing and clinical practice quite another" (1988, p. 41). If Chinese doctors are idiosyncratic, "theirs is no unique condition".

The patient sample

Men predominate in the sample by a proportion of 2:1 (there were 98 men and 49 women). No national figures are kept but this ratio is quite typical of the psychiatric hospitals I have visited in China. Williams & Spitzer (1983) have suggested three types of hypothesis to account for unequal sex ratios. Although their discussion involved depression, their framework applies equally to schizophrenia.

Their first hypothesis is that there may be a difference in true prevalence. However, it is generally accepted that this is not so (Kendell, 1988) although the 1986 epidemiological survey of mental illness in China consistently identified more women than men as suffering from schizophrenia (Co-ordinating Committee, 1986). It seems unlikely that China differs from the rest of the world in this respect, but the issue requires further systematic study to find out whether the difference in China lies in the true prevalence rate, or is being affected by other factors such as inconsistency in diagnostic criteria or inadequate case finding.

Gender differences

It is well known that there are certain differences between men and women in the way that they are affected by schizophrenia. Schizophrenia tends to develop up to six years earlier in men than in women; more women than men suffer their first onset after the age of 40 (Loranger, 1984). Several studies have reported a worse prognosis, at least where hospital discharge rates are concerned, in men than in women (Kendell, 1988). Seeman (1982) reports that women have fewer relapses and are less likely to develop a chronic course. The *International Pilot Study* (Sartorius *et al*, 1986) found female gender to be the best predictor of a remittent (versus chronic) course of illness and one of the five best predictors with respect to the percentage of follow-up time which the patients spent in a psychotic state. Overall, men do not respond as well to psychotropic medication, requiring higher doses of medication, which they do not tolerate as well as women; their long-term adjustment as measured by such indices as social life, marriage, work record, suicide rate and general level of functioning, is not as good as that of women (Torrey, 1988).

To explain these differences, it has been suggested that oestrogen may provide protection through a mechanism not yet understood, or that there may be two different kinds of illness involved, one of which tends to start later and have a more benign course and is prevalent in women; the other to predominate in men, with earlier onset and more damaging long-term effects (Seeman, 1982; Torrey, 1988).

The second hypothesis of Williams & Spitzer (1983) is that psychological variables affect the likelihood of seeking treatment and therefore being entered into the diagnostic data base. While this may be true, the inclusion of only psychological variables is too narrow, when social ones would seem to provide more obvious explanations. This is particularly relevant if what we are trying to account for is an excess of men with schizophrenia who are hospitalised, when there is an excess of women in the clinical population (Co-ordinating Committee, 1986).

The role behaviour associated with being a housewife and mother is possibly easier to carry out than that associated with being a breadwinner, a success in the marketplace. Women's domestic survival skills outside the hospital are likely to be higher than those of men. Given the low rate of marriage among men with schizophrenia (over 60% of the patient sample had never married), once parents die men may have no effective family with whom they can live.

All these reasons probably hold true for the Municipal Hospital sample. In addition, there may be a reluctance to pay for medical care for women on the part of families who will keep them at home rather than pay for expensive treatment. Fewer women have the support of a *danwei* which might be expected to underwrite the cost of medical treatment. One Chinese doctor suggested that one of the reasons for the predominance of male over female in-patients is that women feel a greater sense of responsibility towards parents, husbands and children and are consequently more reluctant to be admitted and tend to stay for shorter periods of time (at least in the acute sector). Men on the other hand, are pleased to be relieved of work and tend to prolong their stays as much as possible.

William & Spitzer's third hypothesis concerns clinician bias in diagnosis. This is not an area that has been researched in China. On what is known, it is possible to argue that women, because they are less associated with violent behaviour, may be more acceptable to families and after-care resources, or are thought to be easier to contain when they are in an excitable or aggressive state.

Age and marital status

The ages of the patients in the sample are quite evenly distributed between the 30s, 40s and 50s, although 60% are over 40 years old. Very few are under 30. This is a predictable picture in a hospital that until recently has accepted very few acutely ill patients and does not have a vigorous discharge policy.

Only 30 of the patients on whom there was information had ever married, and 90 of these patients had never married. Information was unavailable for 27 of the patients.

The people on whom there was no information in the Municipal Hospital sample are the truly sick and destitute for whom there may be a lesser likelihood of marriage. Thus the true 'never married' categories could be higher. This picture is what one would expect based on international data on schizophrenia which shows quite conclusively that patients suffering from this illness have a lower rate of marriage and fertility than in the rest of the population (Kendell, 1988). The difference is more marked among men than among women.

Members of the family of origin are most commonly recorded as next of kin: parents (30%) followed by siblings (20%). This is to be expected given the low rate of marriage among patients. Forty-three per cent of the sample did not have the next of kin recorded on the file. There are two possible reasons for this. Either they have no one who can be named in this category, or the staff, for whatever reason, do not record it. There were a number of instances where some kind of information about a family member carrying out an active role vis à vis the patient was mentioned on the file, even though there was no recorded next of kin. It might also be that, on occasion, a family member accompanying the patient on admission refuses to act as next of kin and to give an address, thus effectively abandoning the patient to the care of the hospital. However, being given as next of kin is no measure of the amount of responsibility taken or care given to a patient. It may simply be someone to inform in the case of death.

Indications of chronicity

The Municipal Hospital opened in 1973. In 1988, the length of current stay of the patient sample (less one missing case) was less than five years for 35.7%; between five and ten years for 20.5%; between ten and fifteen years for 37%; and fifteen years for 6.8%.

For about 12% of the patients their current admission was also their first. Unfortunately, this figure is not wholly reliable as data for 18% of the patients is missing.

The revolving door pattern of admission is common for these patients. At least 87% of them had had previous psychiatric admissions; 15% more than five. The Municipal Hospital was very much a final resting place. For 95% of the sample, their current admission was their first admission to this hospital. All previous admissions had been to hospitals in the acute sector run by the Department of Public Health. Referral to and admission in the Municipal Hospital was a clear indication that the acute sector no longer wished to have anything to do with them, and considered them 'no hopers'. It may be that this happens to them earlier in their psychiatric careers than might have been the case in the UK or USA due to both a lack of community facilities to care for patients who suffer frequent relapses, and a difference in attitudes towards permanent hospitalisation held by medical professionals.

The picture presented is one of chronicity. What is not clear is whether their 'long-stay' character is due to the nature of their illness, the culture and expectations of the hospital, or the paucity of suitable resources and contacts outside it. As previously noted, there has been an admission bulge in recent years in the Municipal Hospital due to an increase in self-pay beds. Will these patients become long-stay because they have been admitted to a hospital that has low expectations about discharge? Would their career have been different if a place had been found for them in the acute sector? Had the acute sector already turned them down as not 'good' enough?

Reasons for admission

Multiple reasons for admission were recorded for many patients. About a quarter were transferred from elsewhere. Very few patients were admitted because they were thought to present a high suicide risk (4.8%). Thirty-four per cent were admitted after acts of aggression, including aggressive acts towards family and non-family. This may be because aggressive behaviour, not well tolerated in China, is more likely to be commented on in the patients' notes and taken as an indication of mental illness.

Relatively lower levels of aggression may provoke a reaction from the Chinese authorities because of high levels of disapproval of such behaviour, which contravenes the norms of social harmony. Related to this are the 30% who were identified as being a threat to public order. This might involve, among other things, disturbing the traffic, annoying the neighbours, setting fire to a house, or destroying property. Some of the events were trivial, others of sufficient severity that they might have led to a criminal charge in the UK. The legal system is much less formalised in China and these incidents were handled by the police, as is permitted, without recourse to the judicial system.

Cultural factors are very much in evidence over admission – as can be seen as a result of the Agricultural Exhibition and in the display of shameless behaviour. Twice a year, in spring and autumn, the local city hosts a particularly substantial Agricultural Exhibition. It is a time when the city authorities want the city to look at its best. Thus 3.4% of the sample was admitted when the police were sweeping the city of vagrants and undesirables because, to quote from one set of casenotes, "the tidiness of the city was being seriously affected". To give this some kind of perspective, *Time* magazine (24 June 1991, p. 45) reported that the Mayor of Atlanta intended to propose an ordinance to outlaw vagrancy (penalty 60 days in prison and/or a $1000 fine). This was because he was concerned that they would create a poor impression on visitors attending the 1996 Olympics.

'Shameless behaviour', for which 15% were admitted, largely covers appearing naked in public, and defecating and urinating in public. Both acts seem intended to shock in a society that is very modest about nudity and bodily functions. There is no dearth of public toilets in the city, where night soil is collected assiduously to supplement scarce agricultural fertiliser. The phrase most commonly used to describe nudity in the casenotes was 'taking off his/her clothes and shamelessly displaying his/her body in public'.

Again it is hard to know whether the occurrence is similar in the UK, but is not regarded as an issue, or whether there is an absolute difference in incidents of public nudity because of different attitudes to public bodily display. If so, this could be related to conservative attitudes towards matters defined as sexual (Ng & Lau, 1990) and reflect the emphasis still placed on propriety (Bodde, 1957).

It also seems that this kind of behaviour has been associated with 'madness' for thousands of years in China. The *Yellow Emperor's Classic of Internal Medicine* cites as one of the symptoms of *kuang* the patient 'always taking off his garments'. Nudity is also mentioned as a symptom by Li (1984), Hsu (1939) and Lamson (1934), who writes about patients taking off their clothes and singing rude songs.

These findings on the prevalence of aggression and behaviour likely to offend against public standards of decency, support observations made in other developing countries. Leff (1988) reports on a study in Swaziland by Guinness that records stripping naked in public as a behaviour associated with psychosis. Gatere in Kenya (reported in Leff, 1988) tried to establish, both among lay people, doctors and traditional healers, the criteria on which they decided that people were mad. The four behaviours on which they agreed, in order of priority, were aggression (particularly attacking people), making a noise, walking naked and talking to oneself.

As Leff points out, in countries where psychiatric facilities are scarce, possibly expensive and where access to treatment may mean a difficult and arduous journey, it is likely that only those patients found to be difficult to manage and very disruptive will be referred. This seems very probable in the Chinese situation where there are few psychiatric beds, so that those likely to be admitted, at least in the past, are those hardest to contain within the community. Behaviour likely to lead to referral comprises violence to people and property and affronts to public decency. Altschuler *et al* (1988), in relation to research that indicated that more manic than depressed patients were admitted to their hospital in China, write:

> "The non-suicidal, withdrawn person is well tolerated in Chinese culture. Conversely, mania is not well tolerated by a community that greatly values conformity and obedience in its members."

This impression is confirmed by Tseng (1973) and K. M. Lin (1981).

In China, as in the UK, care of the sick and handicapped is assumed to be a shared responsibility. In China, the neighbourhood organisation and workplace play a significant role. It is indisputable that the vast majority of people admitted to psychiatric hospital are mentally ill. However not all mentally ill people are admitted to psychiatric hospital, so what sort of events precipitate an admission? It may be a change in the mental state of the patient, but it may also be a change in the caring environment. Thus elderly parents die or a sister marries and there is no one left to care. Or more simply, the family are ground down beyond their limit of tolerance by the patient's behaviour over a period of time. An element of failure in family care was involved in about 26% of the sample reported here. It was also evident that workplace and neighbourhood organisation played little part in sharing the burden of care, judged by the small effect that failure in their involvement had on admissions (6.8%); reaffirming that community care in China means family care.

Information-givers on admission

Another way of looking at this is to examine who provided the information concerning the patient on admission to hospital. The family provided the information in 45% of cases; another hospital's notes were used in 22% of cases. Work colleagues were responsible for escorting 11% of the patients to hospital; neighbourhood cadres were responsible for 4%. This does not signify a major commitment to their care so much as a decision that they are not prepared to take any further responsibility for the patient. Only in 2% of cases was public security responsible for information; in 16% of cases, the source was not known.

Education

Both standard of education and previous employment were routinely included on the admission form in the Municipal Hospital, as is the rule in the rest of China. It was not always possible to tell whether a subject had completed schooling at a particular level, so figures refer to some experience at that level. Because of the nature of the hospital and its prime purpose of caring for the 'three have-nots', it might have been assumed that the standard of education would be very low – this was not the case. In this sample, 43% of the patients had progressed beyond the primary level, 20% had schooling beyond the age of 15, and 5.4% had entered the tertiary level.

The educational level of 30% of the sample is unknown so the figures must be treated with caution. Also, despite the high priority education traditionally is given in China (Bonavia, 1982), all schooling, particularly secondary education, was grossly disrupted during the Cultural Revolution (1966–1976). Schools were closed in 1966; some opened after a year but others remained closed for several more years (Gardiner & Idema, 1973).

China does not appear to publish complete national figures concerning the level of education of the general population, or if so they are not held within the public domain. Such figures may not exist, or the regional and provincial variations may be such as to render them meaningless. What national comparisons can be made that are relevant to the years when many of the patients in the sample would have been at school?

Ensuring that children had access to basic schooling presented many logistical problems because of the size of the population and the scattered nature of the population in rural areas. In 1969 the Draft Programme for Primary and Secondary Education in the Chinese countryside was promulgated. This recommended a system of 5-2-2, or five years in primary school, two years in junior secondary school and two years in senior secondary school. Policy emphasis was placed on completing five years of primary school; while every child was supposed to receive this education, in practice this was difficult to achieve (Bonavia, 1982).

Nearly two-thirds of the sample in the Municipal Hospital had received at least some primary education and most of them had substantially more than that. This represents over 90% when those for whom this data was not known are excluded and compares favourably with what is known of national figures. The *World Bank Report on China* (1986) reports that in 1977, 46% of the eligible age group were enrolled in secondary education (an increase from 2% since 1949). This compares with 42.9% of our sample who had reached that level or beyond, or 61.2% if those for whom data is not available are excluded. The level of illiteracy in the hospital sample is very much lower than the national average of 20.6% (*Beijing Review*, 10 September 1990, p. 18).

Occupation

Occupations in China bear little relation to those used for classification purposes in the West. Three-quarters of the population is classified as rural and works on the land. The majority of town dwellers have little choice about where they work or live since jobs are largely allocated. Most work in factories and relatively few have a professional or managerial post.

In the sample of 147 patients, the occupation of 26 was not known, and 61 had no job at all – in a society where everybody has the right and the duty to work. Some had never had work, particularly those whose age of onset was early. Others had not had a job for many years. Among the women, some had given up work to care for family and children. Twenty-two of the patients were factory workers; 18 were peasants; six had a trade or craft; eight were professionals or managers; and six had other jobs

The relationship between employment status prior to admission and other variables was explored. There was no significant difference between men and women as far as employment history was concerned. Nor was any difference detected on any of the treatment variables, confirming the view that whatever their payment status, patients are treated very much the same.

However, significantly fewer patients who had no job were married (P = <0.0063) and there was a very different profile demonstrated on who had accompanied a patient to the hospital on admission. In comparison with the employed, more unemployed patients were accompanied by relatives as opposed to work unit colleagues; well over half of the unemployed patients were admitted from another hospital or institution, through the public security bureau or neighbourhood office. This suggests a picture of a chronic course of schizophrenia with the concomitant psychosocial deficits that would be very familiar in the West.

It has long been observed in the UK and the USA that more than the expected number of patients with schizophrenia come from the poorest levels of society. Attempts to explain this phenomenon led to the work of Goldberg & Morrison (1964) and Birtchnell (1971) in formulating the concept of 'downward drift' in occupational status. The generally accepted conclusion was that the patients' social status had declined because of the incapacitating effects of the illness, not that poor economic conditions had led to the development of the illness.

To what extent does the concept of 'downward drift' apply in China? The idea is based on the notion that jobs are selected through talent and interest. In China, where jobs are allocated or inherited, they frequently reflect neither. Before the introduction of the contract responsibility system to industry, there was no particular pressure on factories to make a profit. Thus there was little concern about 'carrying' a number of workers, who for a variety of reasons, including mental illness, could not work as well as their colleagues. Now that financial conditions are much more stringent, factories are very reluctant to accept someone, either as a new worker or as a returning worker, whose performance is likely to be erratic. They are also very aware of the high medical bills the work unit will have to pay, another mark against a psychiatric patient.

It is possible that factory workers who become mentally ill may be allocated less responsible, less skilled and consequently less lucrative jobs within the factory. Certainly, this is an issue about which doctors in acute psychiatric hospitals are very concerned. They speak of the difficulties of persuading the patient (on the rare occasions they intervene directly) to accept a drop in status and possibly pay, and of persuading the management to take the worker back and be flexible in job allocation. One way around this that is being explored is the provision of enterprise-based work stations for factory workers suffering from a mental illness (Luo & Yu, 1994). But such facilities are by no means widespread.

In Maoist ideology peasants and workers were at the top of the status pyramid, although matters have altered somewhat in the last ten years. 'Downward drift' in China may lead to unemployability because of the reluctance to employ someone with a psychiatric history, and the lack of alternatives or a free job market. As a concept, it may be too culture-bound to be of any direct relevance in analysing the careers of psychiatric patients in China.

Paying the hospital

The original major purpose of the hospital was to care for the 'three have-nots'. In the sample of 147 patients, 54% were 'three have-nots', while 44% were self-paying. For the total patient population discussed in chapter 5, the figures were 64% 'three have-nots' and 34% self-paying. However, if the sample of patients is divided into those admitted before 1986 and those admitted afterwards, a change of emphasis is seen. In the 1987/88 admission figures, the number of self or *danwei* pay patients has risen to 55% and the 'three have-nots' have fallen to 34%. (The difference between the pre and post 1987 figures was significant at the 0.05 level.) It seems that the original function of the hospital is being clouded by the increased admission of paying patients.

Reasons for onset of illness

Information on the major precipitating factor in the onset of illness in this population was taken from the files (when such reasons were mentioned). A distinction was drawn between a classification of 'not known', in the sense that nothing was mentioned on the file about possible causes of onset (46%), and those cases where the question was asked but no particular reason for onset was discernible (10%). This latter classification would correspond with the concept of insidious onset of schizophrenia.

To a large extent the reasons that are attributed to the onset of schizophrenia are as many and various as they would be in other countries. Most of them are familiar. Work and family stress (14%), problems at school (6%), difficulties with failed personal relationships (9%), are elements of a common human experience. The aspect that is different, and is of great interest to those outside China, is the effect of the Cultural Revolution. Did it cause people to break down? This question is largely unanswerable. Even where it can be shown that some aspect of the Cultural Revolution did have a deleterious effect on a person's mental state, it is impossible to say that the individual would otherwise have remained mentally balanced. Some other, more usual, but none the less very stressful event might have provided a precipitating factor. We can never know.

In the case of the Municipal Hospital sample, a specific event associated with the Cultural Revolution was chosen in that it affected a large proportion of urban young people and many of them found it very distressing indeed: this was the sending of youngsters from the town to villages and communes to learn from the peasants. In only 4% of our sample cases was this policy found to have been involved in schizophrenic onset and it was not found to be significant in the age group affected. When this issue was discussed with staff at the hospital their view was that many people, including themselves, had been 'sent down youth', or in other ways suffered during the Cultural Revolution, without developing major schizophrenic disorder. They concluded that there must have been a pre-existing disposition for schizophrenia to develop.

Available treatments

If genetic and biomedical reasons for illness are the ones most frequently sought by doctors, and if doctors and patients have an expectation that illness is treated by mechanistic means, then it is not surprising that it is the physical treatments from Western medicine that have been adopted into Chinese medicine rather than the psychological ones. Psychopharmacology, hydrotherapy, insulin therapy, prolonged sleep treatment, ECT, and to a lesser extent psychosurgery have all found a welcome place in the repertoire of treatments by Chinese psychiatrists. In addition, from their own repertoire, they have added acupuncture.

Acupuncture, ECT (given unmodified, as is the custom in China) and psychosurgery (20 cases in 1986/87) are part of the treatment regime at the Municipal Hospital. However, the most common kind of treatment is psychopharmacology based on Western drugs. The wide use of such drugs is reported by others (Kao, 1979; Livingstonc & Lowinger, 1983; Young & Chang, 1983, Parry-Jones, 1986), although the range of drugs used may be more restricted.

Cost, of course, is an issue here. All the drugs used at the Municipal Hospital were produced in China and consequently were reasonably priced. A bottle of 100 25 mg tablets of chlorpromazine cost 1.50 yuan. Sometimes patients or their families thought that foreign drugs must automatically be better and were willing to pay considerable amounts for them. China manufactures her own supplies of fluphenazine decanoate which consequently was cheap. However, it did not produce flupenthixol decanoate (at least in 1988) which was imported and consequently cost 66 yuan for 4 cc, or half the local average monthly wage.

The following detailed discussion of drugs in use and prescribing habits is based on information recorded on the current medication cards of the sample of 147 patients at the Municipal Hospital. There is no reason to doubt the accuracy of the information, but it should be remembered that practices in that hospital do not necessarily reflect practices elsewhere.

The range of drugs used is very restricted, consisting of chlorpromazine, perphanazine, trifluoperazine, clozapine, haloperidol and diazepam. There is heavy reliance on two drugs, chlorpromazine and perphenazine. Chlorpromazine is still widely used in the West. It was found to be the most frequently prescribed oral neuroleptic in research carried out in two psychiatric hospitals in Oxford (Michel & Kolakowska, 1981). A study of in- and day patients in a Birmingham psychiatric hospital found that 49.45% of patients were being prescribed either chlorpromazine or haloperidol (Edwards & Kumar, 1984). This compares with 48.97% in this sample. Perphenazine is no longer listed in MIMS (as from April 1989), but was being given to 20% of these patients. Prior to 1990, clozapine was banned in America and restricted in the UK because of the risk of acute agranulocytosis. However, the drug has been available in China for many years and has been widely used; it was being given to 10% of these patients.

No comparative data are available concerning dosage. Dosages tend to be slightly smaller for Chinese patients than for Western patients because of lower body weight. The advice of a lecturer in psychiatry at the Chinese University of Hong Kong was sought in obtaining definitions of low, medium and high dosages for the drugs used in the hospital. With the exception of trifluoperazine – 12 out of the 17 patients receiving it were on a high dose – there was no concentration of patients in the high dosage levels. Most received medium doses.

All drugs being used are recommended by Kendell (1988) to be taken twice daily at 12 hourly intervals; to give them more frequently is an unnecessary imposition.

According to the records available on the 123 patients in the sample taking medication, we found that 101 patients received their medication twice daily; twelve received it three times a day; six received it four times a day; and four received it as required. This compares favourably with Edwards & Kumar's (1984) study where 47% of patients were receiving neuroleptics three or more times a day, suggesting that in this respect the administration of medication is within international standards.

Polypharmacy

Polypharmacy, the concurrent administration to patients of more than one psychotropic drug, is generally not recommended because of increased risk of adverse reactions. There is a lack of evidence for therapeutic advantage from using several psychotropic drugs instead of a properly chosen one; according to Kendell (1988), it is "simply a public display of pharmacological ignorance". Given the sedative properties of neuroleptics, it is hard to justify the concurrent administration of minor tranquillisers and hypnotics (Michel & Kolakowska, 1981). Various studies in the USA, UK, Finland and Israel have shown this to be a problem in both in- and out-patient care (Sheppard *et al*, 1969; Laska *et al*, 1973; Hemminiki, 1977; Schroeder *et al*, 1977; Tyrer, 1978; Yosselson-Superstine *et al*, 1979).

Only 17% of the Municipal Hospital patient sample were in receipt of polypharmacy. Eight patients were taking multiple oral neuroleptics; seven were being given an oral neuroleptic with an anti-cholinergic, and three an oral neuroleptic with a benzo-diazepine, while five were taking all three of these drugs; and two were taking versions of these combinations with multiple oral neuroleptics.

Prescribing habits

The most striking feature in prescribing habits is the lack of use by Municipal Hospital doctors of the injectable depot neuroleptics. Only four cases of their use was recorded in the files. A second feature in the drug regime is that 16% of the sample are on no psychotropic medication at all. A number of interpretations of this phenomenon are possible. Given the hospital's financial dilemma, it might be a cost-cutting exercise. Discussion with the staff suggests that this is probably too cynical a view. Older patients whose symptoms were no longer active were considered not to need to take drugs. No unwillingness to prescribe neuroleptics when it was thought they were needed was observed.

The relatively infrequent use of anti-cholinergic, anti-parkinsonian drugs is notable. In the past these were given routinely, but more recently this practice has fallen into disfavour. It has been found that they alter the absorption of neuroleptics by changes in gut motility, thus reducing the therapeutic action of neuroleptic drugs. They may actually enhance the development of, and obscure the early stages of, tardive dyskinesia. Anti-cholinergic drugs may be abused for their euphoriant effect. Most crucially, patients maintained chronically on anti-parkinsonian drugs and neuroleptics show little increase in side-effects when the former are withdrawn. (Loudon, 1988).

The medical staff at the Municipal Hospital were quite clear that they understood the dangers in the over-prescription of anti-cholinergic drugs, and that clinically they preferred not to use them, unless there was some clear indication that the patient was suffering from side-effects that could not be controlled by an alteration in dosage. Thus in terms of the timing of medication, less multiple drug use, less use of anti-cholinergics, and a high proportion of patients receiving no medication at all, the prescribing habits at the Municipal Hospital conform closely to international standards.

Conclusions

The patients with schizophrenia studied here are predominantly a middle-aged and older population and the figures show clear features of chronicity. Patients have experienced the revolving door phenomenon, but with perhaps not as many revolutions as would be the case in the West, reflecting the greater variety of treatment and rehabilitation modes available in the West. Of concern is the relatively recent phenomenon of admitting paying patients to the Municipal Hospital. They receive the same treatment regime as the other patients and may well become long stay, something that reflects hospital policies rather than the nature of their illness.

The educational level of the patients in the sample compared favourably with what is known of the educational level of China's citizens. The area in which the hospital is situated is one of the more relatively developed areas of China, and one would therefore expect standards to be higher.

The high number of patients who had never worked, or who had been unemployed for a considerable time, was a finding that was not expected. It was not possible to identify the phenomenon of 'downward drift' in this population because jobs in China reflect neither preference nor ability. Patients who had been unemployed before admission were less likely to be married, and much more likely to be admitted through the Public Security Bureau, neighbourhood organisation, or transferred from another hospital or Civil Affairs Bureau reception centre for vagrants.

When precipitating factors at onset were recorded they tended to show the commonality of the human condition: problems at school, in the family, at work, failed relationships with the opposite sex. Although a number of patients had been adversely affected by the events of the Cultural Revolution, there was no evidence, within the age group that would have been most involved, that this was a statistically significant factor in their illness. It is fair to say that on a general level the patients in this sample, as with everyone else in China, have faced levels of hardship and chaos in their lives quite unknown in the UK or the USA.

By the time I had read through 147 case files, a picture formed of a truly 'three have-nots' patient, based on the number of 'no information' boxes ticked on the data collection form. The more that was not known, the more 'have-not' the patient appeared, until it seemed that for some of them only their physical form remained. All else – their personality, their history, their family, their individuality and spirit – had been erased by a combination of their circumstances, their illness and their sojourn in the hospital. There was neither written nor human record of their lives.

7   The patients' voices

Officially, hospitals exist to serve the patients. Patients are the justification for all action taken by the staff and the rationale for the entire organisation; yet such studies as exist of mental hospital services in China say little or nothing about the patients' perspective. Patients exert very little power and their voices go unheard.

To give patients an opportunity to express themselves publicly is difficult. Staff are wary for fear of what might be said about the hospital and the people who work in it. Patients are wary for fear of reprisals from the staff if they speak too freely. Sometimes they have been locked away for so long, and are so institutionalised, that they are not able to express their needs. Sometimes, but by no means as often as one might think, they are deluded and incoherent. None of these factors are sufficient reason for not trying.

Three methods were selected to build as complete a picture as possible about the patients' lives and opinions, chosen because they were achievable. These were data from patients' files, group meetings, and essays written by some of the patients.

Histories of blood and tears

This heading is taken from a comment that a head doctor on one of the male wards made, with some feeling, about the sad and troubled histories of many of the patients on his ward. The phrase stayed in my mind because it expressed a sentiment rarely heard at the hospital. Although the contents of the records are not the authentic voices of the patients, they do provide a sense of both individual experience and how the wider political and social environment impinges on individual lives. The histories are taken verbatim from the files and are presented as found, other than for a little grammatical rearrangement.

Information about the patient's life contained in a file is the product of at least two processes of selection. First, such information is based on interviews with the accompanying relative, or *danwei* representative, not the patient. So material provided relies on what the interviewee knows about the patient, combined with what is thought to be important. Second, out of what is said by the relative, the doctor taking notes is going to select what to 'hear', and what is important or relevant. The resulting story is very much a constructed one.

These are a selection of the more detailed histories and contain the sum total of knowledge remaining about the patients. For many patients, the files contained no background information at all. Comments on files since admission are usually restricted to phrases like 'poor hygiene', 'confused in thinking', 'will answer questions', 'hits and scolds other patients'. There is no further exploration of the self, feelings or experiences. The histories that have been chosen as illustrations have been selected because they are interesting and illuminate common experiences. They do not purport to provide explanations as to why patients became ill, or to be based on a random selection of histories

The women

Ms Wong

Ms Wong has been in hospital at least 11 times. The various hospitals would arrange to discharge her after the Agricultural Exhibition in the spring or autumn, so that there was no longer any danger that she would give a bad impression of the city to visitors. Her misfortunes in life began when she was a child and her parents sold her to an overseas Chinese couple as an adopted daughter. She eventually returned to live with her real mother and started work in a sock factory weaving socks.

She made a free (as opposed to arranged) marriage and at first her marital relationship was good. Her problems started when her husband was sent away to another part of China to work, leaving Ms Wong responsible for four young children and her parents-in-law. In addition to this she had a very poor relationship with her husband's sister.

She started to hear voices and complained that someone put sand in her food. Ms Wong began to assault family members and destroyed furniture at home. All this culminated in her pouring petrol over her sister-in-law's house and attempting to burn it down. She was discovered, restrained and admitted to hospital. The ward notes say that she tends to hit other patients and shouts at them for no reason and describe her as having a 'poor attitude'.

Ms Yip

Ms Yip suffered a high fever when she was 19, while she was being courted by a boyfriend. She began to think about the boy too much, and the ward notes say that the combination of the illness and love affair triggered her first onset of schizophrenia. She received out-patient treatment, and recovered, but had several relapses. When ill she tended to scold heaven, hit other people, damage things and tear up clothes, which she would then mend when she recovered.

Ms Yip married, as she thought, and became pregnant, but since her husband's *danwei* did not approve of the marriage they were not able to go through the official marriage ceremony although they lived together for three years. When she became pregnant the *danwei* leaders forced her to have an abortion at seven months. After that, she and her husband separated. Her mother also suffered from mental illness and was admitted to the city psychiatric hospital run by the Department of Public Health. On one occasion, after discharge, Ms Yip's mother wandered off, did not come back and was never heard from again. So once her father died there was no one to care for Ms Yip. She was having to live on welfare money from the government, and was therefore admitted to this hospital.

Ms Ho

Ms Ho's illness was precipitated when her two children died within quick succession of one another, one from measles and the other from fluid on the lung; and her husband divorced her. She began talking and laughing to herself, behaving bizarrely, drinking dirty water, not eating properly and cutting her clothes down to children's size. Ms Ho had to be looked after by street level cadres, and as she was financially dependent on the government, she was admitted to the hospital.

Ms Lai

Ms Lai became ill in 1966 with no apparent precipitating cause. She talked and giggled to herself and scolded others. She often deliberately harmed herself, beating her own head and chest. Sometimes she cut up clothes with scissors. She broke a window and a water standpipe, and frequently left home for ten days or more without telling anyone where she was going. She would stand in the road and block the traffic. She began to have indiscriminate sexual relations with men and became pregnant twice. The street level association decided that she must have abortions. The patient was not cooperative during the operations and damaged the operating theatre equipment. Her mother died and her father was too old and weak to look after her, so she was sent to this hospital.

Ms Poon

Ms Poon's first episode of illness was in 1960. She married in 1963 and gave birth to a daughter. Then her husband disappeared and deserted her. In order to support herself and the child, she took a job in the market where she met a man with whom she had an affair. Their relationship was discovered when she became pregnant and kept the baby. She was severely criticised by the leaders. She began to sleep all day and wander around at night singing loudly. She also started to assault others. Her file gives no more details, apart from mentioning that her brother also suffered from mental illness.

Ms Kwan

When the Cultural Revolution was at its peak, the class background of Ms Kwan's family was investigated. She found this experience very stressful and became agitated and restless. She burned photographs and her Red Guard sleeve badge on her bed. Gradually, she became more and more withdrawn, refusing to eat or sleep and eventually was admitted to hospital for six months. Since then she has had eight admissions to hospital. Before her last admission to this hospital she became elated and sang lyrics of her own invention constantly, the contents of which were 'low taste and dirty'. She took knives and scissors from her factory which worried other people although she never threatened anyone. Then Ms Kwan went back to her old school, saying that she wished to marry her erstwhile form master. Her family then applied for her to be admitted to this hospital.

The men

Mr Lo

Mr Lo's illness started in the Cultural Revolution, although precipitating factors are not known. It began with him talking to himself, shouting revolutionary slogans, writing big character posters and talking about political matters the content of which was reactionary. He was taken to a psychiatric hospital by officers of the public security bureau and treated for six months. After he was discharged, the patient refused to take medication and his mental state fluctuated. By 1979 he was quite stable, and was given a licence to open a stall in front of the city level Finance Department offices mending metal utensils. When his mental state was unstable he would talk to himself as he sat by his stall, and write big character posters which he would stick on nearby walls, mostly concerning political events that happened in the Cultural Revolution. Mr Lo claimed that people put electricity in him and tried to persecute him. His business was not successful and closed down after several years, mostly because he lost people's pots and pans. After that, he lived on government welfare handouts. Because Mr Lo was acting strangely in front of the Finance Department, it affected the 'tidiness' of the street so the Public Security Bureau brought him to the hospital by force.

Mr So

In 1960, Mr So was sent home to his family from the university where he was studying because they said that he had developed a mental illness, although no details were given. He was admitted to a psychiatric hospital run by the Department of Public Health and, once discharged, worked as a teacher for two months. He could not cope with this job so he went back to live with his parents. Mr So relapsed and was admitted again, and over the next few years was in and out of hospital on at least seven occasions. Eventually, they pronounced him cured and he was sent to a village to work as a teacher; he did this for a year until he relapsed. He was admitted to hospital, treated and sent home.

This time he was sent to a village to work on a farm. He relapsed again, becoming incoherent, shouting reactionary slogans, saying 'down with ...' and naming political leaders at city and provincial levels whom he did not like. He claimed that he was a 'central leader, and that he had authority over the city and district level leaders. Mr So also claimed that he had over 150 mistresses. He was very disturbed at night, shouting and gesticulating. He hit other people and damaged property and then tried to kill himself. He refused drugs, assaulted a female comrade and went into the women's toilet. All in all, his behaviour 'affected social security adversely' and he was admitted to this hospital.

Mr Ma

The origin of Mr Ma's illness is not known but in 1975 his condition deteriorated and he wandered off to the main street, talking incoherently, hitting passers-by, halting traffic. He started fires at home and burned his own clothes and mosquito net. Mr Ma also seriously wounded his father with a kitchen chopper. He wandered the streets begging for food and money, and then assaulted a woman. According to the file "he affected social security with very, very bad consequences". During the Agricultural Exhibition, and at the request of the family, he was admitted through the Public Security Bureau into this hospital.

Mr Keung

During the period before 1949, Mr Keung was a leader of a sabotage unit fighting against both the Guomindang and the Japanese. In 1952 he began to work for the Land Reform movement. In 1953 he fell in love, but the Party objected to the relationship and he started to manifest abnormal behaviour, talking and laughing to himself, failing to look after himself properly. He managed to keep his job until 1960. Then he started to deteriorate further, refusing to bath, picking up food from the streets. However, he did not have his first admission until 1966 when he stayed in hospital for six months. After he was discharged, he refused to take medication and his symptoms returned. For the next 20 years he lived mostly on the streets, wandering from place to place in the city. Once his mother died, he became even worse. As there were no other relatives he became the responsibility of the social security system and, as he was getting old, they decided to admit him here.

Mr Chan

Mr Chan married in 1973. Some time later he began to suspect that his wife was having an affair which led him to request a divorce. Attempts at reconciliation on the part of the *danwei* leaders failed. Soon after the divorce Mr Chan started to behave strangely, crying and laughing loudly, so he was sent for treatment to the Department of Public Health Psychiatric Hospital where he stayed for two years. After discharge, Mr Chan went back to work at his previous *danwei*, where he showed a good attitude towards work and was responsible and efficient. In 1985 the man who lived on the other side of the partition in his room got married. Mr Chan was upset by this and within three days he relapsed, walking about the courtyard at night naked. The case record specifically says that he did not chase women, and also that he still continued to take notice of the *danwei* leader. He was treated at the *danwei* clinic with chlorpromazine.

In 1986 Mr Chan fell in love with a woman who worked in the same *danwei*. He bought her a pot of flowers and wrapped them up in a red cloth on which he had written 'I love you'. The woman refused to accept Mr Chan's gift, and he relapsed again. At this point he was sent back to his village of origin for treatment. Then, without permission, he left his village one day and went back to his work unit to request them to give him back his job. While in the office he began to stare at three women visitors and refused to leave when requested. That night he took off his clothes in public. The *danwei* decided that he could no longer be managed and he was sent to the hospital.

Mr Lau

In 1965 Mr Lau was 'mobilised' as part of the policy to send city youths down to the countryside to learn from the peasants. He had been an apprentice in a factory and was very unwilling to go and work on an orange farm. In 1968 his city residence permit was revoked and, with other city youths, he returned to the city to ask for the permits to be reinstated. This behaviour was strongly disapproved of by one of the local Red Guard factions who chased them.

When Mr Lau returned to his village he was speaking and behaving strangely. He was sent to the local psychiatric hospital for treatment and attacked a doctor. Later, the commune sent him back home to his family, at which time he was demonstrating flat affect and did not want to do anything. He refused to take any advice from his family members. Then he bought cartoon books and stuck them on the wall of his room, and hung posters of women inside his mosquito net. He started to laugh to himself and would cry out 'ghost'! very loudly two or three times in succession. He was admitted and discharged from the Department of Public Health psychiatric hospital three or four times, but would stop taking drugs once at home. After he was discharged in 1982, his family locked him inside the house because he caused such a disturbance in the neighbourhood, throwing rubbish into the next door neighbour's house and destroying property at home. The neighbours complained about him; Mr Lau started to talk about committing suicide, so his family brought him to the Municipal Hospital.

Mr Fung

In 1958, Mr Fung, a city resident, was allocated a job on a farm in Hainan island, at that time a remote and backward area. Initially, his work performance was good, and after work he took an active interest in sports, arts, music and cultural activities. After about two years of working on the farm, he and a female colleague were sent to the city to study. They fell in love, but in 1962 their friendship finished. Mr Fung's behaviour began to change. He started to damage other people's belongings, became hot-tempered and excitable. He talked and laughed to himself and thought that people were trying to harm him. Mr Fung frequently refused to stay in his quarters and would wander off. Often he walked quite far, trying to get back to the city. Whenever he visited his older sister he would scold her. He played with fire and was often involved in criminal damage and assault. Sometimes he was beaten up by others. Mr Fung's behaviour disturbed the neighbours. His illness fluctuated because he would not take medication, although he had been taken to the out-patients department of psychiatric hospitals in the city and Hainan. In 1975 he married a woman from Jiangxi province. However, the marriage only lasted two years because, when she found out that Mr Fung suffered from mental illness, she left him without leaving an address. Their son is now cared for by Mr. Fung's sister.

The group interviews

Two group interviews (one for women and one for men) were held with patients who worked in their ward service groups. Attendance at the interviews was entirely voluntary, thus not all members of the service groups were present. Soft drinks and digestive biscuits were provided as a means of thanking the patients for their cooperation. These group interviews were jointly conducted by two research assistants, who were given guidance as to which areas to attempt to cover, but were asked to encourage the interchange to be as free flowing as possible. The research assistants wrote up their notes of the interviews immediately afterwards and this section is based on their notes. The hospital put no barriers in the way of contact between patients and the research assistants.

The areas that the research assistants were asked to cover with patients were as follows:

Have they been in other hospitals?

How do the hospitals compare?

Are they taking medication?

Do they know what they are taking?

Do they find it helpful?

Have they ever had any other sort of treatment in this hospital or elsewhere?

What sort of things do they do each day?

Are there any special events during the week (e.g. a film night)?

How has the hospital changed since they have lived here?

Is there anything that they would like to see changed?

What is the most memorable thing during their stay in hospital?

Do they still have contact with friends and relatives?

Do they ever think about discharge?

The men

The first group to be held was with male patients. In retrospect, it was agreed that the dynamics of this group were more difficult than those of the female group. A number of factors accounted for this. The two research assistants said that they felt more tense in the male group as it was the first one. At least two patients clearly did not like each other, which led to sharp interchanges and some silences. Two staff members, a nurse and the head doctor from the patients' ward, joined the group after it had begun, and it was also interrupted by the Medical Director coming into the room to 'search for his notebook'.

There was a very dominant member (Mr Lui) whose admiration for the hospital, and constant defence of it, made it difficult for the others to express their opinions freely. Mr Lui was not popular with the other patients, many of whom remained very quiet unless directly addressed. Mr Lui and one other patient were two of the original patients, and had been involved in building the hospital and the holiday camp. The other patients varied in length of admission from six years to six months. The most recently admitted patient said that he had been tricked into coming to the hospital by his relatives, who had told him that they were going to visit a local beauty spot.

The jobs that they do on the ward mainly involve fetching water for collective bathing and ward cleaning. Almost all of them knew what medication they are taking (chlorpromazine), although Mr Lui said that doctors are reluctant to explain anything about medication to the patients. As for special events during the week, they reported that there were none and that in hospital there was nothing memorable to recall.

Many of them had also been in the Department of Public Health hospital at some time in their lives. They did not think that there was much difference between the two in terms of routines, but were agreed that the food in the other hospital was better. One of the patients complained very bitterly about the food once the ward head doctor joined the group, saying that it tasted like grass. Mr Lui became visibly embarrassed and protective of the hospital. Mr Lui felt this hospital had the advantage of having more grounds, as there was no garden at the Department of Public Health psychiatric hospital.

All the patients were single, and five of them were 'three have-nots'. One said that he had lived with his father and sister. Most of the patients said that they wanted to leave but had no plans for the future. One who was a teacher wanted to return to his *danwei*. He had requested discharge for a long time, but had not been granted permission. (It was not clear whether the problem lay with the hospital or the *danwei*.)

Mr Lui had been discharged eight years ago. He enjoyed what was, to the other patients, the very dubious distinction of being the only patient to be discharged from the hospital who had voluntarily requested to come back (because he thought that he was 'getting crazy' again). The other patients made it quite clear that they thought that for this reason, if no other, he was justifiably diagnosed as mad.

Mr Lui described his experiences outside the hospital. For five years after he was discharged, his neighbours called him a 'loonie', and were unpleasant to him. During the last three years this behaviour stopped. He is proud of being the only person ever to ask to come back.

The women

The interview with the women was less constrained. This may have been because there were fewer of them, they were friends, and because this time it was decided to ask staff to leave. Two of the patients were self-pay and one was a 'three have-not'. The first two had been in the hospital for two years and the latter for fifteen – since it opened. All had had experience of the Department of Public Health psychiatric hospital, or its subsidiaries, before coming to the Municipal Hospital. Ms Keung said that she had been tricked into coming to the hospital by the Medical Superintendent and another staff member, who told her that they were taking her to a factory to find work.

All three knew that they were taking chlorpromazine. The doctors told them that they must take it because they were ill, but gave no other explanation. Ms Keung said that she did not like taking medication because, for her, the side effects were very troublesome. Consequently, she had relapsed six times and had spent most of the last ten years in hospital. Sometimes Ms Keung managed to throw her medication away, but if a patient refused drugs, or the staff discovered that they were being thrown away, they would insist that they must be taken. Patients who continued with their 'stubborn refusal', would be held down and the medication forced down their throat.

The patients reported that drugs were the most frequent form of treatment. Sometimes the staff would use electric-acupuncture for 'naughty' patients, although none of them had ever experienced it personally, but had seen it being given. Again, none of them had received ECT but commented that those who had received this treatment said it was very painful.

As service group patients they were expected to work, which in their case meant cleaning, sweeping and washing the rooms of the incontinent patients. Ms Keung said that she would have preferred a lighter job, that she thought there was too much hard work. She would rather do without the one yuan she earned. Ms Han earned 5.50 yuan because she did more work. The 'odd job' nurse used to take them out once a month locally, which they enjoyed, but this had been reduced to every three or four months. They had

had one outing to the city (to the zoo), which they liked even though it was raining.

They commented spontaneously on physical brutality, mentioning particularly one of the domestic workers on their ward, and said that nursing staff sometimes also resorted to physical means of persuasion. They said that at the Department of Public Health psychiatric hospital staff did not hit the patients. Doctors were somewhat different, at least on their ward, where they were kind and showed care and concern for the patients.

They agreed with the men that the food at the Department of Public Health psychiatric hospital was much better. There they had soup twice a week and more variety of vegetables. Here it was mainly vegetable marrow in the summer and cabbage in the winter. Only those on a special diet received soup.

Ms Keung said that there were fights between patients almost every day on the ward, occasionally leading to serious injury. She thought that, if patients were willing to give in, it was possible to avoid fights, especially if they did not care about getting food or medication quickly.

All three patients have relatives. Ms Han's parents were dead but she had five children, some of whom had visited occasionally. Ms Yeung had a father and younger brother but they did not visit. She used to work in a textile factory. Ms Keung used to work as a clerk in the Department of Public Health and her family sometimes took her for home leave. She felt very guilty about placing a burden on the family's finances because they had to pay her hospital fees.

When asked about what changes they would like to see in the hospital, they could not relate this to the ward routines. The only improvement they could think of that had taken place in the hospital was that the appearance of the wards and the gardens over the years had improved. They all wanted to be discharged and go back to work, or in Ms Han's case, to live with one of her children. Ms Keung said that she was ready for discharge and the doctor had given permission. The hospital had written to her father and asked him to take her back, but he had refused. She supposed that this was because she relapsed so frequently.

The essays

I was anxious to reach more of the patients in a way that would permit them to say precisely what they wished, with little outside direction or structure. The original intention of the essay competition that is reported here was to provide all patients with an opportunity, if they wished to take it, to tell something of their lives. The title of the essay ('The Story of My Life') was left deliberately broad so that the patients could choose to write about those aspects which they considered important, without the imposition of someone else's categories or priorities. It also meant that they had the option to reveal or withhold as much or as little as they wished.

It was essential to choose a topic that would not appear threatening in any way to the staff, either professionally or politically. It was made very clear to the staff that patients should not be placed under any duress to participate. In discussion with staff beforehand we asked that they did not influence what patients chose to write about, emphasising that it was important, in order to understand more about the patients, that they were allowed to write what they wished. There were no obvious indications that influence was brought to bear on patients either to include or exclude certain things. However, this fact cannot be guaranteed.

The experiences that are depicted are partly a function of the age of the patients. These were people in their middle years, whose lives had been bisected by the early years of the Communist Government, a variety of political and social upheavals in the 1950s and 1960s, culminating in the Cultural Revolution. Thus their stories reflect the exigencies of the time, for instance the policy of sending urban youth down to the countryside during the Cultural Revolution, or the fact of belonging to or being persecuted by Red Guards.

Such experiences are rapidly becoming history to the younger generation who are too young to remember this period. If we were to perform a similar data collection exercise for those aged between 20 and 35 the themes would be very different. They might, for example, reflect the strain of survival in the new entrepreneurial environment and the problems of adjusting to a social and economic situation that permits choice but expects citizens to exercise more responsibility for themselves in return.

Given that the goal was to find out more about the patients' experience of life the results were somewhat disappointing. Out of 31 entries, 21 were short – fewer than 20 lines. Of these, about seven were very short, of about five lines or fewer. Nine were in the form of, or included, a poem. One was written as a letter to me. Only one was clearly based on fantasy (number 11), and another 3 (numbers 31, 22, 25) (one of which was signed 'Sun Yatsen'), showed evidence of mental confusion. All the rest, even if rather short in some cases, were coherent.

Only ten of the essays contained predominantly personal material that was not wholly centred around life in the hospital, for instance cataloguing schools attended or occupational record. Thirteen of the essays largely centred on matters to do with the hospital, although some of these were personal in the sense that they contained poignant feelings about the individual's situation. One essay in this section (number 23) was entirely devoted to an enthusiastic description of the hospital gardens. Eight of them had nothing to do with the topic at all. Of these, one described the development of construction projects over the last 30 years in the provincial capital (number 30); number 21 was a poem for National Day (October 1., a few days before the competition was held); number 12 was also a poem, this time with no easily described theme; number 18 was largely a description of the hustle and bustle of the local city; number 11 concerned a fantasy about a visit to America as an important diplomat. It was difficult to detect any special theme in numbers 25, 22 and 31. Clearly, for many of them, the story of their lives was the story of their lives in the hospital.

The patients and the party

"We have turned a new page in our lives. Now we can lead a happy life. It is all due to the correct leadership of the government and the Party. I am thankful for the care and concern of the Party with all my heart. I turned out to be nothing even after years of cultivation by the Party. In contrast I became a burden to the country. I feel so ashamed of myself that I want to hide my face. I regretted that I didn't obey the assignment of the Party in the past. If I could work after discharge in the future, I will work hard and listen to the Party, serving the people with all my spirit... In doing so I could pay back the government, the Party and the people for their concern towards me." (A female, divorced parent, *essay 2*)

"The great, glorious and correct Chinese Communist Party, the great People's Republic of China, they loved and cared for the crazy sons and daughters down to the very last detail. They sent the crazy sons and daughters to hospital for treatment." (*Essay 29*, no biographical information)

"I am extremely grateful for the care given to me by the government and I will settle and recuperate without second thoughts." (50-year-old, single male, *essay 3*)

For a Western reader, one of the more surprising features of the essays is the number that include some positive reference to the government and the Party, and a wish to contribute to building socialism in the country, or to contribute to the country generally. Politics is clearly a widely accepted reference point for these patients, whose conception of their government and the Communist Party is a very intimate one.

The immediate analogy that comes to mind is that of a rather authoritarian, but benevolent, parent and a wayward child. The government looks after its citizens in a direct way and in return they are expected to contribute to the development of the country. It may be that because the patient population is predominantly middle-aged, we are dealing either with people who saw the Communist Party make significant gains in improving the quality of the lives of the people; or who went through the period of the Cultural Revolution, where every effort was made to shatter familial identity and replace it with allegiance to the Communist Party. It is impossible to answer the question of whether or not the patients believe in what sounds to a Western ear like political jargon. They may say it because they genuinely believe it, or through intelligent self-interest, or simply out of habit because that is how all people are expected to express themselves.

Attitudes towards the hospital and the staff

"In the hospital doctors and medical staff showed a lot of concern and care...from an unemployed youth, I became part of society. This is inseparable from the concern shown to me by Dr Liang. He showed consideration to me in every aspect. He is really a doctor who treated patients with a parent's heart." (Young man, admitted because of family discord, *essay 17*)

"Celebrate the Number One Education Home
Praise our Motherland
The Number One Education Home changes every day
With green leaves that look like velvet carpets and pavilions
People coming and going. The air is fresh
To build the Number One Education Home as pretty as a picture
Our Motherland will be prosperous and strong"
(*Essay 15*, no biographical information. The Number One Education Home is the old name for the Municipal Hospital)

"I really want to fly over the wall and go back home... I dare not think about my situation. How can I carry on with all this suffering? Alas nobody knows how I feel and understands my sorrow." (A middle-aged female patient, who was one of the original residents transferred from another hospital when this one opened, *essay 5*)

"In the mental hospital doctors and nurses cared for us with serious words and thoughtful hearts. I heard and saw doctors and nurses call out daily 'take your medicine', 'take a bath', 'go to work', 'people upstairs come down to lay the table', 'room check'. Their voices were so cordial. They were really thinking of us." (*Essay 29*, no biographical information)

One-third of the essays either expressed liking for being in the hospital, gratitude towards the staff for the care they were shown, or generally commented on the virtues of the hospital. This is a small number out of a total of 640 and is clearly not random. Even so, in comparison, only two (numbers 5 and 14) showed clear despair or despondency. One interpretation of the positive response to the hospital is that it reflects the level of institutionalisation; that in Goffman's terms, patients are 'converted' (like Mr Lui, see above) or 'colonised'. Yet, it is possible that this is too cynical a view. For those for whom life has been a constant struggle, an organisation that protects, feeds and clothes them may be a preferable alternative to what they have experienced outside the walls. And Mr Lui's evident unpopularity with his fellow patients suggests a certain degree of scepticism among at least some of the others.

The final extract quoted above gives the only example of direct staff–patient communications as patients experience it. The patient uses it as a demonstration of caring. Yet all the phrases are commands and they all express the controlling function of staff over patients' lives. Not one of them is an enquiry into well being, either physical or mental. From a Western point of view this appears significant, but perhaps the meaning is different in the Chinese context.

Hospital conditions and work

"[My job included] cleaning several wards, single rooms, toilets, intensive care unit and drains, etc... I took the broom and several other patients carried water. It was like this every day... It was hard work for me because I was not brought up in a worker's family... At first we were allowed to go out to buy things or to go for a walk with permission; that was a happy thing. But it is not allowed any more. I don't know why. I saw that patients were allowed to smoke in male wards but not female wards. I am not happy at all... I was just being locked up and made to work hard." (*Essay 5*)

"I feel better after coming to the mental hospital. I am not as bad as I was at home. I had a good rest as well. I work in the hospital and feel very happy." (*Essay 9*, no biographical information)

"I joined the service group in the hospital and did cleaning every day which makes me healthy." (*Essay 13*, a homosexual university entrant)

"Life was very simple in the hospital. It was not as good and refined as life at home." (A woman who wishes to observe 'the five standards and the four beauties' – a mass campaign introduced in the early 1980s, targeted at young people, to improve etiquette and public responsibility, *Essay 7*)

"Work includes both mental and physical work. Personally, I think it is more appropriate for mental patients to engage in physical exercise." (*Essay 1*, the only patient to ask to be readmitted)

"On both sides of the path there are many magnolias and you can smell the sweet fragrance of the blooming flowers. There is also a goldfish pond with pretty goldfish in it. It gives the hospital a feeling of tranquillity and elegance." (*Essay 23*, wholly devoted to gardening matters)

"Once you get used to the food in the big cities, I found the food in the Number One Education Institute too bad." (*Essay 27*, referring to a menu from 40 years ago)

Patients rarely commented on the physical conditions of the hospital, possibly because in many ways they were similar to what they had been used to. The selected comments indicate that there is a range of opinion among patients concerning the regime in the hospital. Almost no one mentioned anything to do with direct treatment. What comments there were focused on issues to do with daily occupation, usually in terms of whether or not patients should work and whether, overall, staying in hospital was felt to be beneficial.

Family relationships

"We had three adults in the household and my elder brother was the only breadwinner." (*Essay 28*, a man with a very fractured work record)

"Parents must be very sad when they faced their crazy sons and daughters and found that they were helpless." (*Essay 29*, no biographical information)

"my daughter was seven or eight years old, I couldn't earn enough by just selling junk. Hence I started to beg and sing on the street together with my daughter. When my daughter had reached the age of nine, we started to work as shoe shine and shoe repair workers. In the summer we sold newspapers. Later on I developed a tumour and had to depend on my daughter who carried on our trade repairing and shining shoes and selling newspapers." (Divorced mother, *essay 2*)

"My family haven't visited me. They have not agreed to my discharge... I came from the city but I don't think the leaders here have tried very hard to find out the whereabouts of my family. If only I could go back home I would be grateful." (A middle-aged, female patient, one of the original residents, transferred from another hospital when this one opened, *Essay 5*)

"I feel very sorry that I have been abandoned by people in the community and by my work unit." (*Essay 14*, which expressed much sadness and despair)

Families do not constitute a lively presence in the pages of these essays. They are more remarkable by their absence. This may be accounted for by the many years that patients have remained in hospital; that most of them have had a long history of admissions to hospital, often under circumstances that would have created a burden for families and broken or severely stretched all but the most resilient of family ties; and the remote location of the hospital that made visiting arduous.

The essays indicate that some patients were regretfully aware that they were a drain on family resources in a number of ways. For others the sense of having been abandoned was very acute, made even more so by the realisation that without family support they had very little chance of ever being discharged. For others, for instance the woman who left her husband to live "in love and sweet happiness" with the "most beautiful boy" in the district (*Essay 24*), it is was if the years have not gone by. This woman's hopes of living again with either husband or lover had not faded, even though there had been no contact for many years. There was now probably little apart from dreams to comfort her.

Life before hospital admission

"I became mentally ill when I started university. It was because of homosexuality that has ruined my life and made me spend a long time in hospital." (*Essay 13*)

"[After discharge from the hospital] from a 'loonie' I became a normal person, an editor of the factory newspaper in a printing factory...[to explain the relapse] I had been working continuously for three months, finishing duty after duty, for example preparing for inspection by the deputy mayor, working on the newsletter competition, preparing a bulletin board for festivals, organising a street exhibition, etc. As a result my eating, sleeping and drug taking habits became irregular." (*Essay 1*, the only patient to request re-admission)

"After graduating from teacher training college I was assigned to work as a teacher for two years. I got neurasthenia and the organisation transferred a group of teachers suffering from neurasthenia to another *danwei* to work. I was sent to work as a cashier in a Chinese herbal shop. At that time I was young and would just do things that pleased me. I refused to go as I thought it would be boring sitting down all day. Again I refused to go to work in the New China bookshop because I thought there's nothing technical to learn and the wage was low. And I refused to work in the kindergarten as well. The Education Bureau then transferred me to work as a temporary worker in the street service station. I lost my temporary job after I divorced my husband." (*Essay 2*, a divorced parent)

"The Cultural Revolution started when I was in Form 2 of secondary school. I stopped going to school and stayed at home. Through the neighbourhood committee I worked as a temporary plasterer sometimes. I had not joined any Red Guard organisation. At the age of 18 I joined the call of the country to 'go up to the mountain and down to the village' and joined the Red Army production team of a commune in Hainan Island and participated in the construction of socialism. In 1970, I had an appendectomy in the commune hospital and after the operation had insomnia and was diagnosed as neurasthenic by the doctor. Because I didn't get proper treatment, it developed into mental illness." (*Essay 4*, a male patient whose father was wrongly categorised as a rightist)

Patients' backgrounds are quite varied, and illustrate the ways that larger issues become entangled with individual lives. Many of the patients were 'touched' one way or another by the Cultural Revolution, although not many of them discuss its effects in their essays. The issue of the lack of life choices, particularly over the matter of employment, is very common. The woman quoted in the third extract paid heavily for her intransigence by eventually becoming a street sleeper. Many of the patients were sent from urban to rural areas to work on the communes. Some chose to go, most were forced. All were disrupted.

Hopes for the future

"I want to be discharged soon. After going home, I will obey my father and my mother. I will not hit my grandmother or any one else. I will help my mother and father to do housework and will never go back to the hospital again." (*Essay 20* in its entirety)

"I saw on the television one day that the people and the street office of Xing Guo street organisation take care of the invalids and can make them independent. My suffering is beyond expression when I saw this and compared it with my own dependency. I don't know when I can achieve the goal of being independent. I am not able to discuss this with either the hospital or the work unit. The committee of the work unit don't come to visit me any more... I can only see others' successes with sorrowful eyes. I just wish God would let me die soon." (*Essay 14*, a woman who describes herself as an unwilling invalid because of her illness)

"I am a lunatic. I am very careful at work. I've been waiting a long time for a job." (*Essay 6*, an ex-model worker in a medical machine factory)

"When I am discharged I must treasure my own clothes and not destroy them, or I could give them away generously. If I could be discharged, then from now on I must respect my parents and younger sister. I have to strictly demand myself to have high expectations of myself." (*Essay 7*, the 'five standards and the four beauties')

The future is not the major orientation in these essays. Even those who mention discharge do not look far beyond the moment they are free to walk through the gate. They have been away from the ordinary world too long to be able to conceptualise living in it realistically. Nor do they have access to the knowledge and resources they need to formulate realistic plans.

It is perhaps too much to expect the Municipal Hospital patients to have plans when they are used to having others plan for them, as is the custom, mentally ill or not. Also they know that their fate does not rest in their own hands and is, in a sense, independent of their behaviour, depending as it does on someone else's willingness to look after them and take responsibility for them. Most of them know that realistically there is no one there for them in that respect. Some look back to the past. For others that is too painful. The present, however imperfect, is probably the safest option.

Conclusions

One of the themes that comes out very clearly is how little control people have over the course of their lives, at least in comparison with what would be considered normal in Western countries. Either families or officials make decisions about work, residence, fertility, marriage and opposite sex relationships generally. It is one thing to read about these issues as matters in policy statements, but the histories give us information about the havoc such policies can wreak in individual lives. When one combines this with the deeply institutional nature of the hospital, and the lack of knowledge that patients have about alternatives, it is not surprising that some patients find it hard to think of improvements to the ward routines or think little beyond the day when they are free to leave.

While it is possible that informally in their daily dealings with patients doctors behave differently, what they record in the files shows no psychological insight. The life histories indicate a singular lack of curiosity about clues to the issues that are important for individual patients. The histories sometimes identify areas that one might, in other circumstances, expect to be followed up either overtly in counselling, or at least to inform greater understanding of the individual. Ms Ho, after the death of both her children, begins to cut down her own clothes to children's size. Mr Chan is clearly affected by his inability to establish an emotional and sexual relationship with a woman. But their behaviour is treated wholly as part of their symptomatology, rather than as significant indications to important aspects of inner meaning, which in turn could be useful in the healing process.

With some notable exceptions, patients tended to reveal little of themselves through the essays. Perhaps it was unrealistic to hope that they would. The expression of individuality is not encouraged in China and within the circumstances of the hospital it may well be a protective device to keep feelings locked deeply inside. Others may have been in hospitals for so long that the process of the illness and institutionalisation have gradually erased memory and identity.

There is a very strong emphasis on the will of and control by the Government and Party. While this emphasis on the Government and the Party grates on the Western reader, particularly the patients' tendency to thank the Party and blame themselves, it could also be argued that there is a kind of respect demonstrated in treating psychiatric patients like every one else in terms of political indoctrination, and not using two different standards for the sane and the insane. Normalisation involves replicating conditions for the disadvantaged that bear the closest possible resemblance to normal life. In the Chinese situation, that includes the expectation of making politics part of everyday thinking.

The work ethos is very powerful in China. This is not so much in the expectation to work hard, but that work defines a person and gives access to a social identity and resources that would otherwise be unavailable. Some patients seem to value being able to work in the hospital. Others view it as forced labour. Several of the essays mention a fear of becoming a 'useless person'.

A number of the patients were required to work as virtually unpaid cleaning staff, performing duties like scrubbing out the rooms of incontinent patients, that were not popular with staff. The hospital, if asked, would probably justify it in terms of it being good for the patients' 'rehabilitation', and as a contribution to offset the money that the government is spending to keep them in the hospital. The hospital is there to serve the patients but the patients are there to maintain the hospital.

Many of these patients would not need to be in hospital if community services existed. The evidence from both the essays and the group members indicates that at least some of them are able to work, to think coherently, to write logically. This does not mean that they may not relapse for a time in the future, but the reason that they are in hospital currently does not rest with their mental state, but with the social and family conditions that pertain around them. Their continued incarceration is a product of a lack of supportive and responsive services for both themselves and their families, combined with the policy consequences of resting care solely on the foundation of family, immediately disadvantaging those who are effectively without families.

The question is raised, particularly in the essays, but also to a lesser extent in the groups, as to what extent the patients were self-censoring. They were aware that staff would read the essays and, in the male group, that staff were present. Thus some of the messages may have been for a staff audience. For instance, patients who were promising to respect their parents and not hit family members if discharged, or saying that the food tastes like grass were probably not primarily addressing the research worker!

The more difficult issue for the reader is the temptation to believe the negative things, like the brutality of some of the staff and the misery of some of the patients, because it is what we would expect; to question the genuineness of patients' statements about caring staff or basic contentment with life in the hospital, because to us it seems unlikely. Ultimately, we have to accept what we are told, while constantly bearing in mind that variable opinions are likely; that experiences vary from ward to ward; and that patients in their turn may be using the research process to maximise opportunities to influence their situation.

8   Conclusions

China is changing and, although it would take a brave person to predict future national directions precisely, it does not take a crystal ball to see that the changes are likely to be profound. The ranks of the old guard, survivors of the Long March, are being depleted with the passage of time. The passing of Deng Xiaoping in particular will mark the beginning of a new era; as will the resumption of sovereignty over Hong Kong, the first attempt to meld a vibrant capitalist economy with an ostensibly socialist system, to become 'one country, two systems'. How will this climate of change affect psychiatric care?

Five years on

Five years ago, the Municipal Hospital had no outside phone line; now it does. A donation from a large, local business has enabled it to buy an air-conditioning unit for the meeting room in the administration block. For the staff, both these amenities are symbolic of the hospital entering a more modern age. In 1990, one of the '11 main goals' of the city government was to increase the number of beds in psychiatric hospitals by at least 200, divided between the Civil Affairs and Public Health run institutions. As of 1993, the Municipal Hospital had 800 beds (an increase of 160 since 1988). The expansion was largely paid for by the city government. The staff have interpreted this as a sign that, at long last, the needs of those with a mental illness, and their work with them, are both being given recognition. The numbers of staff have also increased, although the ratio of staff to patients remains virtually the same as in 1988. In 1993, there were two deputy doctors-in-chief, 20 senior doctors and 13 ordinary doctors. The

185

medical staff say that they are beginning to be able to attract new doctors who, having heard good reports about the hospital, wish to work there. In addition to the chief nurse, there are now 60 trained nurses and 101 nursing assistants.

The leaders have three priority areas for developing the hospital. The first is to improve the living conditions of the patients, through renovating the wards and providing more facilities. The second is to improve the management of the hospital, by differentiating treatment regimes more carefully for patients, and through firmer administrative control to cut down on waste and utilise staff in a more rational way. Thirdly, they want to resolve the problem of finding somewhere to discharge rehabilitated patients. To what extent have they been successful in achieving these goals?

Rehabilitation

There has been marked improvement in the facilities available to patients, including the addition of a new rehabilitation building. This contains a well-equipped music therapy room, increasingly popular in China (Tang *et al*, 1994), a recreational activities room, a psychotherapy room, an exercise room and equipment for calligraphy and painting. Doubtless such activities benefit patients, but the number of patients in comparison with the availability of resources does mean that relatively few would be able to participate.

One of the major changes in the hospital has been the addition of two more levels of the treatment programme for male patients, which now includes a rehabilitation ward (52 patients) and a hospital hostel (30 patients). The rehabilitation ward's door is unlocked during the day and patients receive a structured programme centred around work and education sessions regarding aspects of their illness. A considerable amount of money has been spent renovating the ward and buying extra equipment for it, including lockers, tables and chairs. The programme in the ward has been evaluated using a prospective research design and control group. The experimental group (all patients in the ward) showed a significant improvement in overall functioning after a year. The control group (matched patients undergoing standard treatment in the hospital) showed none.

The success of the rehabilitation ward has created a problem for the hospital leaders, as they clearly now have a group of patients whose rehabilitative treatment has been successful and who could move on; only there is nowhere for them to move on to. Their response has been to open a hospital hostel in the grounds. It still has medical and nursing staff on duty but the atmosphere is relaxed and the patients' level of functioning is high. Patients are found work, usually in the hospital or holiday camp, for which they are paid. Opportunities for work in the holiday camp have not been great, and the patients are mostly restricted to 'behind the scenes' functions.

Quality of life

In terms of quality of life, patients in the rehabilitation ward and hostel are very much better off than patients on the ordinary wards. But the hospital leaders realise that they have not solved the major problem: discharge. Their wish is that the work stations could be persuaded to provide residential units, but for reasons discussed earlier, concerning the lack of community acceptance and problems in financing, this is very unlikely to happen.

There have been genuine and significant changes in the hospital, both in terms of resources and regime. The leaders identify at least two issues that they feel remain to be dealt with: poor quality nursing care and the fact that there has not been the same effort to improve and extend the treatment regime among the female patients. Essentially, their situation is much the same as it was in 1988, with two largely undifferentiated wards.

Occupation and time structure

From an outsider's perspective, there is also a continuing difficulty over the question of occupation and time structure for patients. These may be divided into two kinds, the first of which is also perceived by staff. It is very difficult to find sufficient work for the patients on the rehabilitation ward and in the hostel. The reasons behind this are varied. One of them concerns the attitude of people to those with a mental illness. Holiday makers do not want direct contact with them in the holiday camp, partly because they fear it will bring bad luck. Likewise, local farmers have been very reluctant to hire the rehabilitated patients as farm labourers. In addition, hospital staff are, perforce, taking up the role of entrepreneur, looking for secondary processing work (like packaging) that can be done by patients and that requires minimal equipment. This depends on having the right contacts in the manufacturing sector, not generally thought to be a prerequisite for medical staff! They are handicapped in this respect by being located in a primarily agricultural area, with little significant local industry. If the work is found in the city, then that brings transportation complications. In addition, the availability of such work is subject to the 'boom and bust' nature of the Chinese economy. All in all, it is not surprising that the staff experience quite some difficulties in this area.

However, there is another aspect to occupation. For those patients who are not on the rehabilitation ward or in the hostel, there still seems to be a paucity of daily activity. The staff have a very narrow definition of occupation. For them it means work and if there is none to be had, or the patient is not sufficiently able, that tends to be the end of the story. Training in the skills of daily living and recreational activity on a daily basis involving interaction between staff and patients still does not happen. A non-governmental organisation, based in Hong Kong and specialising in the care of those who have had a mental illness, is co-ordinating a project that will work with nursing staff at the hospital to provide them with skills training appropriate to working with long-stay patients. The hospital leaders are supportive of this scheme but it remains to be seen how effective it will be.

Future challenges for psychiatry in China

Psychiatric care in China has developed in response to three political imperatives: every citizen must contribute their labour to socialist construction; disruptive behaviour must be controlled; and the state and community must employ the principle of constructing a 'socialist spiritual civilisation' to provide services for those with a disability (Phillips & Pearson, 1994). Such instructions do not provide sufficient guidance to persons working in the field, many of them without training. The lack of psychological and sociological perspectives on ways of caring for people with a mental illness has severely restricted the possibility of developing indigenous models of biopsychosocial care that are based on scientific principles and rigorous research. A number of challenges remain to be faced.

The need for public education

Whatever changes take place, they will occur in an environment that is essentially hostile to people with a mental illness and their needs; a problem China shares with other countries, including the UK (*Community Care*, 26 August 1993, pp. 12–13), but which in China is particularly pervasive. Attempting to persuade a population to be more accepting of those with severe mental disorders is notoriously difficult but until the level of stigma attached to mental illness in Chinese society is reduced, the difficulties in developing community-based services are unlikely to be overcome. Of particular importance is the fact that many people required to work with those with a mental illness have little training to prepare them for this work, and they frequently share all the same prejudices as the lay person. This not only includes Department of Civil Affairs cadres, and staff and volunteers in work stations, but also doctors and nurses. While the task of educating the general public is an overwhelming one, targeting those who work with mentally ill people would be much more achievable. In addition, advantage could also be taken of the state's control of the media to introduce accurate and sympathetic portrayals of those with a mental illness in popular 'soap operas'. State control over the school curriculum could be used in the same way. Fundamental changes in attitude will not be wrought overnight but opportunities to promote change that could be utilised without major resource implications exist, and these could be pursued more vigorously.

Training and motivation

Currently, most of the people who work with those suffering from a mental illness either have no training at all for the jobs they do, or, in the case of qualified doctors and nurses, a training that is profoundly biological in orientation with very little or no psychiatric content. Thus there are two problems. The first is to disseminate what knowledge there is to people who need it, and the second is to improve and make more relevant the existing stock of knowledge.

The lack of social sciences teaching in medical and nursing training has severely curtailed the development of well-grounded models of non-biologically-based intervention strategies. Social sciences (particularly sociology and psychology) are once more being taught in universities. However, as medical universities are traditionally separate entities, the potential for social sciences to cross over into the medical and nursing curricula may be limited.

In particular, there is a need for social sciences knowledge in the area of psychosocial treatment and rehabilitation, important in both community and hospital settings. Related to this is the potential for nurses to take up more active and challenging roles as therapists and as community mental health workers. Current activities of nurses are largely concerned with looking after the physical needs of patients and controlling them, neither of which are particularly satisfying activities. Improving training, increasing skill level and making the job more inherently satisfying would perhaps also have the knock-on effect of increasing motivation and job status.

There still remains the issue of introducing different kinds of workers into psychiatric care. It will be a long time before social work, occupational therapy and clinical psychology gain a secure foothold within the range of mental health professionals. However, as part of the new emphasis on people with a disability, a new post of 'rehabilitation worker' has been designated by the State Personnel Bureau. Such an addition to recognised positions is difficult to achieve, but has the advantage of conferring official recognition, a job description and a place in the pecking order. Rehabilitation workers are designated to work with those with physical disabilities, but lobbying from influential psychiatrists might lead to the inclusion of a psychiatric component in their training, and placement in psychiatric settings.

Financing psychiatric services

The single most important factor that will affect the shape of psychiatric services in China in the short and medium term is the issue of financing. Both hospital and community-based services are increasingly expected to be largely self-financing. This has forced many enterprises, including hospitals, to try and run successful businesses on the side to subsidise their welfare services. Such activities, particularly if they are successful, can come to dominate the attention and interest of the cadres involved, to the extent that the welfare services are neglected (Wong, 1994). Nor do all cadres or hospital officials have the skills and talents to be entrepreneurs, in which case they may add to their burdens worries about unsuccessful business ventures.

The most obvious result of this new emphasis on self-sufficiency is the increase in hospital fees. Another change in policy, that has permitted the opening of private institutions, is almost certainly going to lead to a proliferation of poor quality 'hospitals', where the fees will deliberately undercut those of rivals run by the Departments of Civil Affairs or Public Health. Even so, it will still fall largely to families to pay for treatment out of their own pockets, a burden that many will still not be able to afford.

One way around this, of course, would be to follow what the World Bank's report on China (1992) suggests as a general principle: to increase ambulatory care. There are already at least two successful projects in rural China that utilise this idea, in

Shandong and Sichuan provinces. But part of their success comes from the fact that they receive training input from psychiatrists based in hospitals. Doctors are becoming increasingly reluctant to participate in schemes whose success reduces the income from fees to hospitals, on which the specialists' salaries are dependent! There is, of course, no reason why in the new economic climate, the hospitals should continue to effectively subsidise home-bed schemes. A more realistic charge could be levied on the family, something which would almost certainly be cheaper than hospital care. The success of such schemes depends on a significant number of staff being willing to leave the comfort and security of their hospitals and go out into the community. It is conceivable that this could happen in urban areas, but in rural areas the reluctance of qualified, higher level doctors to work in the countryside, particularly in the remoter parts, would still need to be overcome.

Community based care

Care outside the hospital would seem preferable for most patients on a number of grounds: it is cheaper, more convenient, less disruptive of ordinary life and potentially less damaging. But what does care consist of? Currently, according to the government's own reports, the majority of people with a mental illness do not receive appropriate treatment of any kind. It would be a great achievement to be able to deliver basic psychopharmacological care to them on a regular and reliable basis.

But beyond that, what else is there? For many patients, only the family is there to provide emotional support and negotiate the difficult hurdles of work and marriage. Little has been done to identify the family as the major caring resource for psychiatric patients in China, and to devise policies that will strengthen and support them in their efforts. A form of family intervention, started in Hubei province, and designed with the conditions in China in mind, has been shown in an evaluative study lasting two years to reduce the number of admissions of the patient to hospital, and to reduce the period between admissions (Xiong *et al*, in press). This is clearly of both therapeutic and economic benefit to the family and patient. In the current economic climate, it may not be such good news to the hospital because it reduces the potential source of income from admissions. The invisibility of the family as a resource to be nurtured is demonstrated in the '64 sites' project described earlier. This is by far the most comprehensive statement on community-based care for psychiatric patients

ever made in China; and here the family is mentioned neither as
a resource nor as a target of care.

A further difficulty is that two of the most significant aspects of
China's community care programme, guardianship networks and
work stations, rely heavily on volunteers. Volunteers are usually
older women, with a low level of education, who are frequently
accused of acting as agents for the government (Chan, 1993). This
obviously raises questions about the standard of services provided,
although such a method of service provision is entirely coherent
with the CCP's long-standing emphasis on grassroots involvement
and anti-professional stance. However, yet again, the era of
economic reform casts shadows over the continuation of the spirit
of voluntarism. On the whole, the traditional group from which
volunteers are drawn is becoming more interested in finding a
way to supplement their pensions, or availing themselves of the
greater opportunities for recreational activities.

Administration and co-ordination

Economic reform has meant a greater decentralisation down to
provincial and municipal areas, and with it a concomitant loss of
control by the central government. Policy formulation has always
been a top–down process in China, but when the government
does not have the money to back up the implementation of its
policies, the chances of change occurring are greatly reduced.
The Beijing authorities are reduced to a 'leading and guiding'
role. While there is plenty of room for 'grassroots–up' initiatives
in the realm of psychiatric care, they rely very much on individual
enthusiasm. Sadly, with such a devalued client group, this
enthusiasm is rare. Effectively, this leaves a vacuum where initiative
and implementation ought to be.

There are also problems in co-ordination between and within
bureaucracies. China's enormous size both in terms of geography
and population means that the vertical links in government
departments are sorely stretched. They have to take account of the
fact that what makes sense in Sichuan may have little relevance in
Xinjiang. If vertical links are problematic, horizontal links between
bureaucracies, in this case government departments, are almost
non-existent. This is why the government places so much emphasis
on the 'three man leading groups', consisting of representatives
of the departments most involved in providing services for those
with a mental illness, in an attempt to create such linkages. Direct
observation suggests that co-operation is most successful when it is
based on *guanxi* and is thus personal and idiosyncratic. Again, it

is significant that the '64 sites' plan does not consider the issue of how the services are going to be co-ordinated and how a network of services might be developed. Wang (1994) demonstrates how a network can be developed which permits patients to move easily between the various services as their needs change. But it is significant that she remains in charge of the whole operation and that it is self-financing. Thus inter-bureaucracy liaison becomes unnecessary.

The involvement of Deng Xiaoping's son, Deng Pufang, in the area of welfare for disabled people has done much to galvanise a previously moribund situation. Lobbying by senior psychiatrists to have psychiatric rehabilitation included under this rubric was an inspired move. Deng Pufang has the power and connections to ensure that the various ministries work together. Whether this momentum can be sustained depends on two things: that of Deng Pufang maintaining influence in his own right after the death of his father; and psychiatric rehabilitation continuing to be accepted as part of the movement to help the disabled, even though it does not produce the startling results that are sometimes obtainable through physical treatments, for example, cataract operations.

Does ideology matter?

Anyone who knows about psychiatric care in Western countries will have recognised sadly familiar aspects of psychiatric care in China, but there are also major differences. The interests of the individual are given less emphasis in China than the rights of the collective. There are fewer community support services for both patients and their families. There is much less understanding and acceptance among workers in psychiatric settings of the social and emotional difficulties that contribute to the onset and maintenance of illness. Overall, China has fewer resources at its disposal to spend on mentally ill people.

Nonetheless, there is still the question of why there are so many similarities in attitude and treatment of mentally ill people in China and the West. The answer almost certainly lies in the nature of the disorder under discussion and societal reaction to it.

Sarbin & Mancuso (1980) claim that rather than being a medical diagnosis, schizophrenia is a moral verdict. In reality, it is both. The handicaps of schizophrenia lie not only in the disease but in other people's reactions to it. The symptoms are frightening to many when in their florid form, and frequently take the shape of flouting concepts of public propriety. Although episodes of violence are not particularly common, they are common enough to create what feels like a realistic fear to bystanders. Status in any community is founded on the individual's ability to perform in appropriate age and sex-related roles, maintain standards of propriety and modesty, and behave appropriately in kinship and social interaction. It is exactly in these areas that people with severe mental disorders do not conform. Failure to conform to these expectations will almost certainly lead to a social devaluation of the person concerned.

Barham makes the point that all of us have to answer the question 'who am I?' as a more or less continuous (and changing) process throughout our lives. To do this, we are involved in constructing a narrative of our lives which, because it has to take into account other peoples' narratives as they interweave with our own, can never be fully predictable.

Whatever the nationality, the patient with schizophrenia has to construct a narrative for the future with a devalued identity, that takes into account others' hostile reactions and a future that is unpredictable at best.

> "If I become a useless person after going into mental hospital then all my hopes and expectations will be dreams." (*Essay 5*)

This excerpt from one of the patients' essays expresses very well the restraints that are placed on the narrative future by becoming redefined as a 'useless person'. Barham (1984, p. 184) describes a very similar feeling among the patients in his study:

> "Among schizophrenic people, loss of confidence in the viability and value of their life projects, and the reconstruction of themselves as useless, are as much as anything powerful determinants in the transformation of a potentially manageable disability into permanent social disablement and chronicity, and adverse secondary reactions like these are fuelled and aggravated by forms of contextual disadvantage such as unfavourable attitudes and expectations of others, lack of opportunity to practice social skills, isolation from everyday life and enforced pauperism."

Thus both in China and in Western countries, the terms of participation in social life which someone who suffers from schizophrenia is permitted, are defined by others. It is not simply a question of setting a 'mental hospital', with its connotations of degradation, against the 'community', embodying beneficence. Indeed, the concept of community as a site is not helpful. What is really under discussion is not the question of distance or proximity but the idea of a moral community, based on respect for the more vulnerable members of society, and of the sorts of policies and practices that might be constructed in order to enhance the terms of participation in social life for such people. The issue is not whether people live in hospital or outside it, but how they might come to live a valued life.

At the heart of the similarities in attitude toward people with schizophrenia in China and elsewhere, is convergence of the negativity of the moral verdict and the resultant exclusion from the moral community and a valued life. The form of moral community and the content of a valued life are immaterial. The defining feature is to be excluded from them. Thus the universal reaction to schizophrenic disorder is almost always negative, superseding factors like political philosophy or available economic resources.

In turn, this negative reaction colours the way that the distribution of available resources takes place. It is true that the UK and USA have greater disposable national incomes, so that facilities for mentally ill people are generally more diverse and of better quality than in China. But comparisons of priorities within each country would show that mentally ill people are worse off in relation to other groups.

How significant is the economic and political context in which psychiatric care takes place?

> "Some of the most basic needs of the mentally disabled, above all the needs for housing, for occupation and for community are not satisfied by the market system of resource allocation under capitalism... The crisis of mental health provision...is simply the crisis of the normal social order in relation to any of its members who lack the wage based ticket of entry into its palace of commodities." (Sedgwick, 1982, p. 239)

But does the socialist system, or at least the version of it pertaining in China, do any better? China has substituted the *danwei* for wages but the effect is much the same.

It is very difficult to sustain a thesis that socialism, because of its different economic substructure, produces a political and cultural superstructure that, in its emphasis on the grassroots and mass participation, produces an environment which is more accepting of people with a mental illness. They are placed low in lists of priorities the world over. Individual political systems are irrelevant – our tasks, if not necessarily our solutions, are held in common.

Bibliographies

Sources in English

ACHTENBERG, H. (1983) Mental health care in China. *Journal of Psychiatric Treatment and Evaluation*, **5**, 371–375.

ADAMS, F. (1972) Mental care in Peking. *China Now*, January.

ALABASTER, E. (1899) *Notes and Commentaries On Chinese Law*. London: Luzac.

ALTSCHULER, L. L., WANG, X., QI, H. Q., *et al* (1988) Who seeks mental health care in China? Diagnoses of Chinese outpatients according to DSM–III criteria and the Chinese classification system. *American Journal of Psychiatry*, **145**, 872–875.

BAKER, H. D. R. (1979) *Chinese Family and Kinship*. London: Macmillan.

BANISTER, J. (1987) *China's Changing Population*. California: Stanford University Press.

BARHAM, P. (1984) *Schizophrenia and Human Value*. Oxford: Basil Blackwell.

BAUM, R. (1986) Modernization and legal reform in post-Mao China. *Studies in Comparative Communism*, **19**, 69–103.

BIRTCHNELL, J. (1971) Social class, parental social class, and social mobility in psychiatric patients and general population controls. In *Aspects of the Epidemiology of Mental Illness* (ed J. A. Baldwin), pp. 77–103. Boston: Harvard University Press.

BLOOMINGDALE, L. M. (1980) Chinese psychiatry after Mao Zedong. *Psychiatric Annals*, **10**, 7–24.

BODDE, D. (1957) *China's Cultural Tradition*. Hinsdale, Ill: Dryden Press.

—— (1980) Age, youth and infirmity in the law of Ching China. In *Essays on China's Legal Tradition*, (eds J. A. Cohen, R. R. Edwards & F. M. C. Chen), pp. 137–169. Princeton, NJ: Princeton University Press.

BONAVIA, D. (1982) *The Chinese: A Portrait*. London: Pelican.

BOWMAN, K. M. (1948) Psychiatry in China. *American Journal of Psychiatry*, **105**, 70–71.

BRAYFIELD, J. (1978) Psychiatric care. *Social Work Today* (Birmingham), **10**, 24.

BREGER, E. (1984) A child psychiatrist's observation on care of the mentally ill in the People's Republic of China. *Psychiatric Hospital*, **15**, 3, 127–132.

BROWN, L. B. (1980) A psychologist's perspective on psychiatry in China. *Australian and New Zealand Journal of Psychiatry*, **14**, 21–35.

—— (1981) *Psychology in Contemporary China*. London: Pergamon Press.

—— (1983) Social psychiatry in China. *British Journal of Social Psychiatry*, **22**, 363–372.

BUEBER, M. (1992) Letter from China (No. 1). *Archives of General Nursing*, **vi**, 61–64.
—— (1993*a*) Letter from China (No. 2). *Archives of General Nursing*, **vii**, 111–115.
—— (1993*b*) Letter from China (No. 3). *Archives of General Nursing*, **vii**, 249–253.
—— (1993*c*) Letter from China (No. 4). *Archives of General Nursing*, **vii**, 311–316.
BUNGER, K. (1950) The punishment of Chinese lunatics and negligents according to the classical Chinese law. *Studia Serica*, **9**, 1–16.
BURCH, B. B. (1979) Models as agents of change in China. In *Value Change In Chinese Society* (eds R. W. Wilson, A. A. Wilson & S. L. Greenblatt), pp. 122–140. New York: Praeger.
CERNY, J. (1965) Chinese psychiatry. *International Journal of Psychiatry*, **1**, 229–247.
CHAO, Y. C. (1965) Neurology, neurosurgery and psychiatry in new China. *Chinese Medical Journal*, **84**, 714–742.
CHAN, C. L. W. (1993) *The Myth of Neighbourhood Mutual Help: The Contemporary Chinese Community Based Welfare System in Guangzhou*. Hong Kong: Hong Kong University Press.
—— & CHOW, N. W. S. (1992) *More Welfare After Economic Reform? Welfare Development in the People's Republic of China*. Hong Kong: Centre of Urban Planning and Environmental Management, The University of Hong Kong.
CHEN, P. C. & TUAN, C. H. (1983) Primary health care in rural China: post-1978 development. *Social Science and Medicine*, **17**, 1411–1417.
CHEUNG, P. (1991) Adult psychiatric epidemiology in China in the 1980s. *Culture, Medicine and Psychiatry*, **15**, 479–496.
CHIN, R. & CHIN, A. (1969) *Psychological Research in Communist China* 1949–1966. Cambridge, MA: MIT Press.
CHINA LAW YEAR BOOK (1989) (eds The Publishing House of Law, Beijing). London: Butterworth's Press.
CHISWICK, D. (1988) Forensic psychiatry. In *Companion to Psychiatric Studies* (4th edn)(eds R. E. Kendell & A. K. Zealley), pp. 660–681. Edinburgh: Churchill Livingstone.
CHIU, M. L. (1981) Insanity in imperial China: a legal case study. In *Normal and Abnormal Behaviour in Chinese Societies* (eds A. Kleinman & T. Y. Lin), pp. 75–94. Dordrecht: D. Reidel.
CHOW, N. W. S. (1987) Western and Chinese ideas of social welfare. *International Social Work*, **30**, 31–41.
—— (1988) *The Administration and Financing of Social Security in China*. Hong Kong: Centre of Asian Studies, Hong Kong University.
—— (1994) *Social Security Reform In China: An Attempt To Build Up A Socialist Social Security System With Chinese Characteristics*. Monograph 4, Social Welfare in China Series. Hong Kong: Department of Social Work and Social Administration, Hong Kong University.
COHEN, D. (1989) *Soviet Psychiatry*. London: Paladin.
COHEN, J. A. & GELATT, T. A. (1984) *The Criminal Law and the Criminal Procedure Law of China*. Beijing: Foreign Languages Press.
CONNER, A. (1993) Commentary: amendments to the Chinese constitution. *Hong Kong Law Journal*, **23**, Part 2, 224–226.
COPPER, J. F., MICHAEL, F. & WU, Y. L. (1985) *Human Rights in Post-Mao China*. Boulder, CA: Westview Press.
CRANSTON, M. (1973) *What Are Human Rights?* London: The Bodley Head.
CROIZIER, R. (1975) Medicine and modernization in China: an historical overview. In *Comparative Studies of Health Care in Chinese and Other Societies* (eds A. Kleinman & P. Kunstadter). Washington, DC: US Department of Health, Education and Welfare.
CUI, N. F. (1988) Reflections on a social security system with Chinese characteristics. *International Social Security Review*, **2**, 171–175.

DAES, E-I. (1986) *Principles, Guidelines and Guarantees For The Protection of Persons Detained On Grounds of Mental Ill-health or Suffering From Mental Disorder*. New York: United Nations.

DEAR, M. (1984) Health services planning: searching for solutions in well-defined places. In *Planning and Analysis in Health Care Systems* (ed. M. Clarke), pp. 7–21. London: Pion.

DIEN, S. F. D. (1983) Big me and little me: a Chinese perspective on self. *Psychiatry*, **46**, 281–287.

DIXON, J. (1981) *The Chinese Welfare System*. New York: Praeger.

EDWARDS, S. & KUMAR, V. (1984) A survey of prescribing psychotropic drugs in a Birmingham hospital. *British Journal of Psychiatry*, **145**, 502–507.

FALLOON, I. R. H., BOYD, J. L., McGILL, C. W., *et al* (1985) Family management in the prevention of morbidity in schizophrenia. *Archives of General Psychiatry*, **42**, 887–896.

FREARS, M. (1976) Fighting for freedom: mental health care in China. *Rehabilitation World*, **2**, 21–22.

GARDINER, J. & IDEMA, W. (1973) China's educational revolution. In *Authority, Participation and Cultural Change in China* (ed. S. Schram), pp. 257–287. London: Cambridge University Press.

GOLDBERG, E. M. & MORRISON, S. L. (1963) Schizophrenia and social class. *British Journal of Psychiatry*, **109**, 785–802.

GOSTIN, L. (1987) Human rights in mental health: a proposal for five international standards based upon the Japanese experience. *International Journal of Law and Psychiatry*, **10**, 353–368.

GU, X., BLOOM, G., TANG, S., *et al* (1993) Financing health care in rural China: preliminary report of a nationwide study. *Social Science and Medicine*, **36**, 385–391.

HANSEN, C. (1985) Punishment and dignity in China. In *Individualism and Holism: Studies in Confucian and Taoist Thought* (ed. D. Munro). Ann Arbor, MI: Centre for Chinese Studies, The University of Michigan.

HARRIS, M. (1979) *Cultural Materialism*. New York: Random House.

—— (1987) *Cultural Anthropology* (2nd edn). New York: Harper & Row.

HART, H. L. A. (1968) *Punishment and Responsibility; Essays In The Philosophy of Law*. Oxford: Clarendon Press.

HEGINBOTHAM, C. (1987) *The Rights of Mentally Ill People*. London: Minority Rights Group.

HEMMINIKI, E. (1977) Polypharmacy amongst psychiatric patients. *Acta Psychiatrica Scandinavica*, **56**, 347–356.

HENDERSON, G. (1990) Increased inequality in health care. In *Chinese Society On The Eve of Tiananmen; The Impact of Reform* (eds D. Davis & E. Vogel). Cambridge, MA: Harvard University Press.

—— & COHEN, M. (1984) *The Chinese Hospital: The Socialist Work Unit*. New Haven: Yale University Press.

HIGGINS, J. (1981) *States of Welfare: Comparative Analysis in Social Policy*. Oxford: Basil Blackwell.

—— (1986) Comparative social policy. *The Quarterly Journal of Social Affairs*, **2**, 221–242.

HILLIER, S. M. (1988) Health and medicine in the 1980s. In *Reforming the Revolution: China in Transition* (eds R. Benewick & P. Wingrove) London: Macmillan.

—— & Jewell, J. A. (1983) *Health Care and Traditional Medicine in China 1800–1982*. London: Routledge and Kegan Paul.

HO, D. Y. F. (1974) Prevention and treatment of mental illness in the People's Republic of China. *American Journal of Orthopsychiatry*, **44**, 621–636.

HSU, F. L. K. (1939) A brief report on the police co- operation in connection with mental cases in Peiping. In *Social and Psychological Studies in Neuro-Psychiatry* (eds R. Lyman, V. Maguer & P. Liang) Beijing: Henri Vetch.

—— (1985) The self in cross-cultural perspective. In *Culture and Self; Asian and Western Perspectives* (eds A. J. Marsella, D. Devos & F. L. K. Hsu), pp. 24–55. New York: Tavistock

HUMAN RIGHTS IN CHINA (1991) Beijing: Information Office of the State Council.

INGRAM, J. H. (1918) The pitiable condition of the insane in north China. *The China Medical Journal*, **32**, 134–135.

JABLENSKY, A. (1988) Epidemiology of schizophrenia. In *Schizophrenia: the Major Issues* (eds P. Bebbington & P. McGuffin), pp. 19–35. Oxford: Heinemann.

JIANG, Z. N. (1988) Community psychiatry in China: organisation and characteristics. *International Journal of Mental Health*, **16**, 30–42.

JIN, D. X. & Li, G. S. (1994) The role of human rights and personal dignity in the rehabilitation of chronic psychiatric patients: a rural therapeutic community in Yanbian, Jilin. *British Journal of Psychiatry*, **165** (suppl. 24), 121–127.

KAMENKA, E. (1978) The anatomy of an idea. In *Human Rights* (eds E. Kamenka & A. Tay), pp. 1–12. London: Edward Arnold.

KAO, J. J. (1974) Psychiatry in the People's Republic Of China: a prospectus. *American Journal of Chinese Medicine*, **2**, 441–444.

—— (1979) *Three Millenia of Chinese Psychiatry*. New York: Institute for Advanced Research in Asian Science & Medicine Monograph Series.

KARENGA, M. R. (1978) Chinese psycho-social therapy; strategic model for mental health. *Psychotherapy Theory, Research and Practice*, **15**, 101–107.

KENDELL, R. F. (1988) Schizophrenia. In *Companion to Psychiatric Studies* (4th edn), (eds R. E. Kendell & A. F. Zealley), pp. 310–334. Edinburgh: Churchill Livingstone.

KENT, A. (1993) *Between Freedom and Subsistence: China and Human Rights*. Hong Kong: Oxford University Press.

KERR, J. G. (1898) The refuge for the insane, Canton. *The China Medical Missionary Journal*, **12**, 177–178.

KETY, S. S. (1976) Psychiatric concepts and treatment in China. *China Quarterly*, **66**, 315–323.

KINCHELOE, M. (1985) A glimpse of psychiatric nursing in China. *Vermont Registered Nurse*, April, pp. 3, 4, 12, 14.

KING, A. & BOND, M. (1985) The Confucian paradigm of man: a sociological view. In *Chinese Culture and Mental Health* (eds W. S. Tseng & D. Wu). Orlando: Academic Press.

KLEINMAN, A. (1986) *Social Origins of Distress and Disease: Depression, Neurasthenia, and Pain in Modern China*. New Haven: Yale University Press.

—— (1988) A window on mental health in China. *Scientific American*, **76**, 27.

—— & LIN, T. Y. (1981) *Normal and Abnormal Behaviour in Chinese Culture*. Dordrecht: D. Reidel.

—— & MECHANIC, D. (1979) Some observations of mental illness and its treatment in the People's Republic Of China. *Journal of Nervous and Mental Disease*, **17**, 267–274.

KRAFT, A. M. & SWIFT, S. S. (1979) Impressions of Chinese psychiatry, December 1978. *Psychiatric Quarterly*, **51**, 83–91.

KUIPERS, L. (1991) Schizophrenia and the family. *International Review of Psychiatry*, **3**, 105–117.

LAMPTON, D. M. (1977) *The Politics of Medicine in China – The Policy Process 1949–1977*. Folkestone: Western Press/Dawson & Sons.

LAMSON, H. D. (1935) *Social Pathology in China*. Shanghai: The Commercial Press.

LASKA, E., VARGA, E., WANDERLING, J., et al (1973) Patterns of psychotropic drug use for schizophrenia. *Diseases of the Nervous System*, **34**, 294–305.

LAU, C. C. (1993) The Chinese family and gender roles in transition. In *China Review, 1993* (eds J. Y. C. & M. Brosseau), pp. 20.1–20.18. Hong Kong: Chinese University Press.

LAWYERS' COMMITTEE FOR HUMAN RIGHTS (1993) *Criminal Justice with Chinese Characteristics: China's Criminal Process and Violations of Human Rights*. New York: Lawyers' Committee for Human Rights.

LAZURE, D. (1964) Politics and mental health in New China. *American Journal Of Orthopsychiatry*, **34**, 925–933.

LEFF, J. (1988) *Psychiatry Around the Globe* (2nd edn). London: Gaskell.

——, BERKOWITZ, N., SHAVITZ, et al (1989) A trial of family therapy v. a relatives group for schizophrenia. *British Journal of Psychiatry*, **154**, 58–66.

LEFLEY, H. P. (1986) Why cross cultural training? Applied issues in culture and mental health service delivery. In *Cross Cultural Training for Mental Health Professionals* (eds H. LeFley & P. Pederson). Springfield, Ill: Thomas.

LENG, S. C. & CHIU, H. D. *Criminal Justice in Post-Mao China; Analysis and Documents*. Albany: State University of New York Press.

LEUNG, S., et al (1978) Chinese approach to mental health service. *Canadian Psychiatric Association Journal*, **23**, 354–359.

LI, S. X. & PHILLIPS, M. R. (1990) Witchdoctors and mental illness in mainland China. *American Journal of Psychiatry*, **147**, 221–224.

LI, Z. Z. (1984) Traditional Chinese concepts of mental health. *Journal of the American Medical Association*, **252**, 3169.

LIN, K. M. (1981) Traditional Chinese medical beliefs and their relevance for mental illness and psychiatry. In *Normal and Abnormal Behaviour in Chinese Society* (eds A. Kleinman & T. Y. Lin), pp. 99–114. Dordrecht: D. Reidel.

LIN, N. (1988) Chinese family structure and Chinese society. *Bulletin of the Institute of Ethnology Academica Sinica*, **65**, 59–129.

LIN, T. Y. (1983) Psychiatry and Chinese culture. *Western Journal of Medicine*, **139**, 862–867.

—— (1984) A global view of mental health. *American Journal of Orthopsychiatry*, **54**, 369–374.

—— (1985) Mental disorders and psychiatry in Chinese culture: characteristic features and major issues. In *Chinese Culture and Mental Health* (eds W. S. Tseng & D. Wu), pp. 369–394. Orlando: Academic Press.

—— (1985*a*) The shaping of Chinese psychiatry. In *Mental Health Planning For One Billion People; A Chinese Perspective* (eds T. Y. Lin & L. Eisenberg), pp. 3–37. Vancouver: University of British Columbia Press.

—— & EISENBERG, L. (1985) *Mental Health Planning For One Billion People*. Vancouver: University of British Columbia Press.

—— & LIN, M. C. (1981) Love, denial and rejection: responses of Chinese families to mental illness. In *Normal and Abnormal Behaviour in Chinese Societies* (eds A. Kleinman & T. Y. Lin), pp. 387–402. Dordrecht: D. Reidel.

LIU, J. H. & JIA, J. T. (1994) Medicine and the law in the People's Republic of China. Paper presented at the Taniguchi Foundation Nineteenth International Symposium, Division of Medical History. September 4–10, Fuji Institute of Education and Training, Shizuoka, Japan.

LIU, X. H. (1980) Mental health work in Sichuan. *British Journal of Psychiatry*, **137**, 371–376.

—— (1981) Psychiatry in traditional Chinese medicine. *British Journal of Psychiatry*, **138**, 429–433.

—— (1983) Psychiatry. In *Modern Chinese Medicine* Vol. 2, (ed. H. G. Wu). MTP Press.

LIVINGSTONE, M. & LOWINGER, P. (1983) *The Minds of the Chinese People*. Englewood Cliffs, NJ: USA.

LORANGER, A. W. (1984) Sex difference in age of onset of schizophrenia. *Archives of General Psychiatry*, **41**, 157–161.

LOUDON, J. B. (1988) Drug treatments. In *Companion to Psychiatric Studies* (4th edn), (eds R. E. Kendell & A. K. Zealley), pp.682–708. Edinburgh: Churchill Livingstone.

Lu, Y. C. (1978) The collective approach to psychiatric practice in the People's Republic of China. *Social Problems*, **26**, 2–14.

Lucas, A. (1982) *Chinese Medical Modernization; Comparative Policy Continuities, 1930s–1980s.* New York: Praeger.

Luo, K. L. & Yu, D. S. (1994) Enterprise based sheltered workshops in Nanjing: a new model for the community rehabilitation of mentally ill workers. *British Journal of Psychiatry*, **165** (Suppl. 24), 89–95.

Lyman, R. S. (1937) Psychiatry in China. *Archives of Neurology and Psychiatry*, 765–771.

——, et al (1939) *Neuropsychiatry in China.* Peking: Henri Vetch.

Madsen, R. (1984) *Morality and Power in a Chinese Village.* Berkeley, CA: University of California Press.

Masserman, J. H. (1980) Psychiatry in China: background, theory and practice. *Current Psychiatric Therapies*, 195–206.

McCartney, J. L. (1926) Neuropsychiatry in China; a preliminary observation. *Chinese Medical Journal*, **40**, 617–626.

Medvedev, Z. & Medvedev, R. (1971) *A Question of Madness.* London: Penguin.

Michel, K. & Kolakowska, T. (1981) A survey of prescribing psychotropic drugs in two psychiatric hospitals. *British Journal of Psychiatry*, **138**, 217–221.

Minogue, K. R. (1978) Natural rights, ideology and the game of life. In *Human Rights* (eds E. Kamenka & A. Tay) London: Edward Arnold.

Mishra, R. (1981) *Society and Social Policy; Theories and Practice of Welfare* (2nd edn). London: Macmillan.

Munro, D. (ed.) (1985) *Individualism and Holism: Studies in Confucian and Taoist Thought.* Ann Arbor: Center for Chinese Studies, University of Michigan.

Nathan, A. (1986*a*) Political rights in Chinese constitutions. In *Human Rights in Contemporary China* (eds R. Randle Edwards, L. Henkin & A. J. Nathan), pp. 77–124. New York: Columbia University Press.

—— (1986*b*) Sources of Chinese rights thinking. In *Human Rights in Contemporary China* (eds R. Randle Edwards, L. Henkin & A. J. Nathan), pp. 125–165. New York: Columbia University Press.

—— (1994) Human rights in Chinese foreign policy. *The China Quarterly*, **139**, 622–625.

Needham, J. (1970) *Clerks and Craftsman in China and the West.* Cambridge: Cambridge University Press.

Ng, M. L. & Lau, M. P., (1990) Sexual attitudes in the Chinese. *Archives of Sexual Behaviour*, **19**, 373–388.

Ng, V. W. (1980) Ching laws concerning the insane: an historical survey. *Ching Shi Wen Ti*, **4**, 55–89.

—— (1991) *Madness In Late Imperial China.* Norman, Oklahoma: University of Oklahoma Press.

Palmer, M. (1986) Family law in the People's Republic of China. *Journal of Family Law*, **25**, 41–68.

Parry-Jones, W. Ll. (1986) Psychiatry in the People's Republic of China. *British Journal of Psychiatry*, **148**, 632–641.

Pearson, V. (1989) Making a virtue of necessity: hospital and community care for the mentally ill in China. *International Social Work*, **32**, 53–63.

—— (1989) Law and the mentally ill in the People's Republic of China. *International Bulletin of Law and Mental Health*, **1**, 3.

—— (1991) The development of modern psychiatric services in China 1898–1949. *History of Psychiatry*, **ii**, 133–147.

—— (1992*a*) Community and culture: a Chinese model of community care for the mentally ill. *The International Journal of Social Psychiatry*, **38**, 163–178.

—— (1992*b*) Law, rights and psychiatry in the People's Republic of China. *International Journal of Law and Psychiatry*, **15**, 409–423.

—— (1993) Families in China: an undervalued resource for mental health? *Journal of Family Therapy*, **15**, 163–186.

—— (1995a) Health and responsibility: but whose? In *Social Change and Social Policy in Contemporary China* (eds L. Wong & S. MacPherson). Basingstoke: Avebury Press (in press).

—— (1995b) In search of quality; population policy and eugenics in China. *British Journal of Psychiatry* (in press).

—— & Jin, D. (1992) The view from below: the experience of psychiatric consumers in China. *Asia-Pacific Journal of Social Work*, **2**, 45–55.

—— & Phillips, M. R. (1994a) Psychiatric social work and socialism: problems and prospects in China. *Social Work*, **39**, 280–287.

—— & —— (1994b) The social context of psychiatric rehabilitation in China. *British Journal of Psychiatry*, **165** (Suppl. 24), 11–18.

PEAY, J. (1989) *Tribunals on Trial*. Oxford: Clarendon Press.

PERRING, C., TWIGG, J. & AITKEN, K. (1990) *Families Caring for People Diagnosed as Mentally Ill; The Literature Re-examined*. London: Her Majesty's Stationery Office.

PHILLIPS, M. R. (1993) Strategies used by Chinese families in coping with schizophrenia. In *Chinese Families in the 1980s* (eds D. Davis & S. Harrell). Berkeley and Los Angeles, CA: University of California Press.

—— & PEARSON, V. (1994) Future opportunities and challenges for the development of psychiatric rehabilitation in China. *British Journal of Psychiatry*, **165** (Suppl. 24), 128–142.

——, —— & Wang, R. W. (1994) *Psychiatric Rehabilitation in China. Models for Change in a Changing Society*. British Journal of Psychiatry, **165** (Suppl. 24).

PINKER, R. (1985) Social policy and social care: divisions of social responsibility. In *Support Networks in a Caring Community* (eds J. A. Jonker & R. A. B. Leaper). Dordrecht: Martinus Nijhoff.

PRIEMUS-NOACH, M. (1988) Mental health in China; notes and impressions. *China Information*, **3**, 55–63.

PRINS, H. (1980) *Offenders, Deviants or Patients?* London: Tavistock.

PYE, L. (1988) *The Mandarin and the Cadre; China's Political Cultures*. Ann Arbor, MA: University of Michigan Press.

QIU, F. & LIU, S. Q. (1994) Guardianship networks for rural psychiatric patients: a non-professional support system in Jinshan County, Shanghai. *British Journal of Psychiatry*, **165** (Suppl. 24), 114–120.

RATNER, C. (1979) Mental illness in the People's Republic of China. *Voices*, **14**, 80–84.

ROSE, R. & SHIRATORI, R. (1986) *Welfare States East and West*. Oxford: Oxford University Press.

ROSNER, S. (1976) Treatment in China. *Mental Hygiene*, **60**, 5–9.

SAINSBURY, M. J. (1974) Psychiatry in the People's Republic of China. *Medical Journal of Australia*, **1**, 669–675.

SARBIN, T. T. & MANCUSO, J. C. (1980) *Schizophrenia. Medical Diagnosis or Moral Verdict?* New York: Pergamon.

SARTORIUS, N., JABLENSKY, A., KORTEN, G., *et al* (1986) Early manifestations and first contact incidence of schizophrenia in different cultures. *Psychological Medicine*, **16**, 909–928.

SCHROEDER, N. H., CAFFEY, E. M. & LOREI, T. W. (1977) Antipsychotic drug use: physician prescribing practices with psychotherapeutic drugs. *Archives of General Psychiatry*, **35**, 1271–1275.

SEDGWICK, P. (1982) *Psycho Politics*. New York: Harper & Row.

SEEMAN, M. V. Gender differences in schizophrenia. *Canadian Journal of Psychiatry*, **27**, 107–112.

SELDEN, C. (1905) Work amongst the Chinese insane and some of its results. *The Chinese Medical Missionary Journal*, **19**, 1–17.

—— (1908) The John G. Kerr Refuge for the Insane. *The China Medical Journal*, **22**, 82–91.

—— (1909) Treatment of the insane; Parts 1 & 2. *The China Medical Journal*, **23**, 221–233 & 373–385.

—— (1937) The story of the John G. Kerr Hospital for the Insane. *Chinese Medical Journal*, **52**, 704–714.

SHEN, Y. C. (1983) Community mental health care within primary care in the People's Republic Of China: the home care program in the Beijing countryside. *International Journal of Mental Health*, **12**, 123–131.

—— (1985) Community mental health home-care programme, Haidian District in the suburbs of Beijing. In *Psychiatry, The State of the Art: Epidemiology and Community Psychiatry*, **7**, pp. 423–428. New York: Plenum Press.

SHEPHERD, G. (1991) Psychiatric rehabilitation for the 1990s. In *Theory and Practice of Psychiatric Rehabilitation* (2nd edn) (eds F. N. Watts & D. H. Bennett), pp. xiii–xivii. Chichester: Wiley.

SHEPPARD, C., COLLINS, L., FIORENTINO, D., *et al* (1969) Polypharmacy in psychiatric treatment; incidence at a state hospital. *Current Therapeutic Research*, **11**, 765–774.

SIDEL, R. (1973) The role of revolutionary optimism in the treatment of mental illness in the People's Republic of China. *American Journal of Orthopsychiatry*, **43**, 732–736.

—— & Sidel, V. (1973) *To Serve The People; Observations on Medicine in the People's Republic of China*. New York: The Josiah Macey Foundation.

—— & —— (1982) *The Health of China*. London: Zed Publications.

SIU, Y. M. & LI, S. M. (1993) Population mobility in the 1980s: China on the road to an open society. In *China Review*, 1993 (eds J. Y. S. Chen & M. Brosseau), pp. 19.1–19.31. Hong Kong: The Chinese University of Hong Kong.

SPENCE, J. (1980) *To Change China; Western Advisers in China 1620–1960* (2nd edn). New York: Penguin.

TANG, W. Z., YAO X. W. & ZHENG, L. P. (1994) Rehabilitative effect of music therapy for residual schizophrenia: a one-month randomised controlled study in Beijing. *British Journal of Psychiatry*, **165** (Suppl. 24), 38–44.

TAO, J. (1990) The Chinese moral ethos and the concept of individual rights. *Journal of Applied Philosophy*, **7**, 119–127.

TARRIER, N., BARROWCLOUGH, C., VAUGHN, C., *et al* (1988) The community management of schizophrenia: a controlled trial of a behavioural intervention with families to reduce relapse. *British Journal of Psychiatry*, **153**, 532–542.

TAY, A. E. S. (1978) Marxism, socialism and human rights. In *Human Rights* (eds E. Kamenka & A. E. S. Tay). London: Edward Arnold.

THOMPSON, R. K. C., MCKENZIE, W. & PEART, A. F. W. (1967) A visit to the People's Republic of China. *Canadian Medical Association Journal*, **97**, 349–360.

THORNICROFT, G. (1987) Contemporary psychiatry in China. *International Journal of Mental Health*, **16**, 86–94.

TIAN, W. C., PEARSON, V., WANG, R. W., *et al* (1994) A brief history of the development of rehabilitative services in China. *British Journal of Psychiatry*, **165** (Suppl. 24), 19–27.

TI'EN, J. K. (1985) Traditional Chinese beliefs and attitudes towards mental illness. In *Chinese Culture and Mental Health* (eds W. S. Tseng & D. Wu), pp. 67–82. New York: Academic Press.

TORREY, E. F. (1988) *Surviving Schizophrenia; A Family Manual* (2nd edn). New York: Harper & Row.

TOUSLEY, M. M. (1985) China: psychiatric nursing in the People's Republic. *Journal of Psychosocial Nursing and Mental Health Services*, **23**, 28–35.

TSENG, W. S. (1973) The development of psychiatric concepts in traditional Chinese medicine. *Archives of General Psychiatry*, **29**, 569–577.

TUCKER, S. (1983) *The Canton Hospital and Medicine in 19th Century China (1835–1900)*. Ann Arbor, MI: University Microfilm International.

TYRER, P. (1978) Drug treatment of psychiatric patients in general practice. *British Medical Journal*, ii, 1008–1010.

VISHER, J. S. & VISHER, E. B. (1979) Impressions of psychiatric problems and their management: China, 1977. *American Journal of Psychiatry*, **136**, 28–32.

WALDER, A. G. (1986) *Communist Neo-Traditionalism; Work and Authority in Chinese Industry*. Berkeley, CA: University of California Press.

WALLS, P.D., WALLS, L.H. & LANGSLEY, D.G. (1975) Psychiatric training and practice in the People's Republic of China. *American Journal of Psychiatry*, **132**, 121–128.

WANG, G. W. (1979) *Power, Rights and Duties in Chinese History. The Fortieth George Ernest Morrison Lecture in Ethnology*. Canberra: Australian National University.

WANG, Q. T., GONG, Y. Z. & NIU, K. Z. (1994) The Yantai model of community care for rural psychiatric patients. *British Journal of Psychiatry*, **165** (Suppl. 24), 107–113.

WANG, X. S. (1994) An integrated system of community services for the rehabilitation of chronic psychiatric patients in Shenyang, China. *British Journal of Psychiatry*, **165** (Suppl. 24), 80–88.

WANSBOROUGH, N. (1981) The place of work in rehabilitation. In *Handbook of Psychiatric Rehabilitation Practice* (eds J. Wing & B. Morris), pp. 79–94. Oxford: Oxford University Press.

WATTS, F. & BENNETT, D. H. (1981) Introduction: the concept of rehabilitation. In *Theory and Practice of Psychiatric Rehabilitation* (eds F. N. Watts & D. H. Bennett), pp. 3–14. Chichester: Wiley.

WEI, X. W. (1988) Social security system in mainland China. Paper presented at the Seminar on Social Work Education in the Asian and Pacific Region, held in Beijing.

WILLIAMS, J. B. W. & SPITZER, R. L. (1983) The issue of sex bias in DSM–III; a critique of *A Woman's View of DSM–III* by Marie Kaplan. *American Psychologist*, **38**, 793–798.

WILSON, H. S. & HUTCHINSON, S. A. (1983) Nursing in China: three perspectives – psychiatric diagnoses range from depression and violence to social and sexual nonconformity. *American Journal of Nursing*, **83**, 393–395.

WING, J. K. (1978) *Reasoning about Madness*. Oxford: Oxford University Press.

WONG, K. C. (1950) A short history of psychiatry and mental health in China. *Chinese Medical Journal*, **68**, 44–48.

WONG, L. (1992) Community social services in the People's Republic of China. *International Social Work*, **35**, 455–470.

—— (1993) Slighting the needy? Social welfare under transition. In *China Review, 1993* (eds J. Y. S. Cheng & M. Brosseau). Hong Kong: Chinese University Press.

—— (1994) Privatisation of social welfare in post-Mao China. *Asian Survey*, **34**, 307–325.

—— & MACQUARRIE, L. (1986) *China's Welfare System; A View From Guangzhou*. Hong Kong: Hong Kong Polytechnic.

WOODS, A. H. (1929) The nervous diseases of the Chinese. *Archives of Neurology and Psychiatry*, **21**, 547–570.

WORLD BANK (1984) *Report on China*. Washington: The World Bank.

—— (1989) *World Development Report, 1989*. Washington: The World Bank.

—— (1992) *China: Long-Term Issues and Options in the Health Transition*. Washington: The World Bank.

WORLD HEALTH ORGANIZATION (1973) *The International Pilot Study of Schizophrenia*. Geneva: WHO.

—— (1979) *Schizophrenia: An International Follow-Up Study*. Chichester: Wiley.

WU, C. (1959) New China's achievements in psychiatry. In *Collection of Theses on Achievements in the Medical Science in Commemoration of the Tenth National Foundation Day of China*, **2**, Beijing. Translated by US Joint Publications Research Service, No.14, 829, p. 601.

XIA, Z. Y. & YAN, H. Q. (1980) Mental health work in Shanghai. *Chinese Medical Journal*, **93**, 127–129.
——, —— & Wang, C. H. (1987) Mental health care in Shanghai. *International Journal of Mental Health*, **16**, 81–85.
—— & Zhang, M. Y. (1981) History and present status of modern psychiatry in China. *Chinese Medical Journal*, **94**, 277–282.
XIONG, W., PHILLIPS, M. R. & WANG, R. W. (1994) Family-based intervention for schizophrenic patients in China: a randomized controlled trial. *British Journal of Psychiatry*, **165**, 239–247.
YAN, S. M., CHEN, D. Y., CHAO, Y. Z., *et al* (1982) Prevalence and characteristics of mania in Chinese inpatients: a prospective study. *American Journal of Psychiatry*, **139**, 1150–1153.
——, *et al* (1984) The frequency of major psychiatric disorder in Chinese inpatients. *American Journal of Psychiatry*, **141**, 690–692.
—— & XIANG, D. H. (1984) Psychiatric care in the People's Republic of China. *IRCS Medical Science–Biochemistry*, **12**, 193–194.
YANG, K. S. (1986) Chinese personality and its change. In *The Psychology of the Chinese People* (ed. M. Bond), pp. 106–170. Hong Kong: Oxford University Press.
YAO, C. Y. (1985) Mental health in primary care in Yantai prefecture: a rural model. In *Mental Health Planning for One Billion People* (eds T. Y. Lin & L. Eisenberg). Vancouver: University of British Columbia Press.
YOUNG, D. & CHANG, M. Y. (1983) Psychiatry in the Peoples' Republic of China. *Comprehensive Psychiatry*, **24**, 431–438.
—— & XIAO, M. Y. (1993) Several theoretical topics in neurosis research. *Integrative Psychiatry*, **9**, 5–12.
YOSSELSON-SUPERSTINE, S., STERNIK, D. & LIEBENZON, D. (1979) Prescribing patterns in psychiatric hospitals in Israel. *Acta Psychiatrica Scandinavica*, **37**, 504–509.
ZHANG, M. L., WANG, M. T. & LI, J. J. (1994) Randomised control trial of family intervention for 78 first episode schizophrenic patients: an 18-month study in Suzhou, Jiangsu. *British Journal of Psychiatry*, **165** (Suppl. 24), 96–102.
ZHANG M. Y., YAN, H. Q. & PHILLIPS, M. R. (1994) Community-based psychiatric rehabilitation in Shanghai: facilities, services, outcome and culture specific characteristics. *British Journal of Psychiatry*, **165** (Suppl. 24), 70–79.
Zhi, M. (1991) Pre-marital check-ups in China. *Women in China*, January, 18–19.
ZHU, N. S., Ling, Z. H., Shen, J., *et al* (1989) Factors associated with the decline of the co-operative medical system and barefoot doctors in rural China. *Bulletin of the World Health Organization*, **67**, 431–441.

Sources in Chinese

BEIJING MEDICAL UNIVERSITY (ed) (1986) *Medical Psychiatry and Related Problems*. Vol. 3. Changsha: Hunan Science and Technology Publishing House.
CHEN, D. Y., YAN, X. M. & CHAO, Y. C. (1984) The application of the Chinese diagnostic criteria: a comparison with DSM–III. *Chinese Journal of Neurology and Psychiatry*, **17**, 90–92.
CO-ORDINATING GROUP FOR THE 12 REGION EPIDEMIOLOGICAL STUDY OF MENTAL ILLNESS (1986) Investigation of the prevalence of various mental disorders and analysis of the data. *Chinese Journal of Neurology and Psychiatry*, **19**, 80–82.
FANG, Y. Z. , ZHANG, Y. J., GUO, B. H., *et al* (1982) A survey of marital state and family planning of schizophrenics. *Chinese Journal of Neurology and Psychiatry*, **15**, 204–206.
GUAN, X. (1988) The science of forensic psychiatry from two murder cases. *Law Science Monthly*, **80**, 38–39.
GUO, J. Y. (1987) *Forensic Medicine*. Beijing: People's Health Publisher.

206   *Mental Health Care in China*

JIA, Y. C. (1983) Forensic psychiatry; questions and answers. *Jurisprudence*, **25**, 36–37.

LI, C. P., LI, Y. Z., LIU, P. Z., *et al* (1987) Case analysis of schizophrenics by the psychiatric expert testimonial service. *Chinese Journal of Neurology and Psychiatry*, **20**, 135–138.

MO, G. M. (1959) The achievements of the Guangzhou City Mental Hospital over ten years. *Chinese Journal of Neurology and Psychiatry*, **5**, 310–311.

PHILLIPS, M. R., XIONG, W. & ZHAO, Z. A. (1990) *Issues Related to the Use of Assessment Instruments for Negative–Positive Psychiatric Symptoms*. Hubei: Science and Technology Press.

REN, G. J. (1988) *A General Survey of Marriage Law*. Beijing: Chinese University of Politics and Law Press.

SHEN, Y. C. (1958) Prevention and treatment of mental illness should use politics first policy and go the people's way. *Chinese Journal of Neurology and Psychiatry*, **5**, 347–350.

SUN, J. W. (1984) Schizophrenic homicide – report of six cases. *Chinese Journal of Neurology and Psychiatry*, **17**, 140–142.

SUN, K. J., WANG, W. & YE, C. S.(1987) *Concise Dictionary of Civil Affairs*. Sichuan, Chengdu: Sichuan Science and Technology Publishing House.

WU, J. S. (1985) A brief discussion of the ability of mentally ill patients to take responsibility for their illegal acts and offences. *Law Science Monthly*, **44**, 43–45.

WU, X. C. (1983) A study of schizophrenics with criminal behaviour as the characteristic feature. *Chinese Journal of Neurology and Psychology*, **16**, 338–339.

XUN, M. L. (1986) The problem of birth control in schizophrenic patients. *Chinese Journal of Neurology and Psychiatry*, **19**, 335–338.

YU, D. J. (1987) Legal bases for forensic psychiatry; a discussion of the fifteenth clause of the penal code of China. *Chinese Journal of Neurology and Psychiatry*, **20**, 132–134.

YUAN, T. G. & PENG, C. X. (1987) The transformation of the schizophrenic subtypes in the last twenty years. *Chinese Journal of Neurology and Psychiatry*, **20**, 340–343.

ZHANG, D. J. (1987) The speech of the vice minister of civil affairs in the second national health conference. *Selected Documents in Civil Affairs Work*, pp. 249–256. Beijing: Huaxia Chubanshe.

ZHANG, H. (1987) A commentary on the principles of jurisprudence in forensic psychiatry. *Chinese Journal of Neurology and Psychiatry*, **20**, 129–131.

ZHONG, X. S. & SHI, Y. Q. (1987) A preliminary analysis of 210 cases for forensic psychiatric appraisal. *Chinese Journal of Neurology and Psychiatry*, **20**, 139–141.

ZUTANGSHAN EDUCATION AND REARING HOSPITAL (1958) How does the Zutangshan Education and Rearing Hospital manage mental patients? *Chinese Journal of Neurology and Psychiatry*, **4**, 259–262.

Index

Compiled by CAROLINE SHEARD

Tang Code 31–2
therapy
  Chinese medicine 27–8
  post 1980 27–8, 121
  pre-1949 12
  principles 18, 132
  psychosocial, five point model 22–5
'three have-nots' 161
  health services for 75–6
  in Municipal Hospital 116–17, 120–1
  welfare services for 64–5
'three man leading groups' 69–70, 192
'three pardonables' 31
  townships 73
  training 12, 76–8, 121–2, 189–90
    Mao Zedong's directive on 77
    nursing staff 82, 122–3, 189–90
    postgraduate specialist 78–80
  trifluoperazine 159
  Twelve Regions Survey 67–8
  urban areas
    health insurance 71–3
    and health policy 91
    migration of skilled health personnel to 79
  village doctors 74, 80–1
  vomiting induced by herbal medicine 28
  welfare factories 65–6
  welfare mix 62
  welfare services 61–2
    and the family 62–3
    state provision 64–6
    workplace 63–4
  Western visitors, during Cultural Revolution 20–1
  work therapy stations 106–8, 192
  workplace 92, 102
    and welfare provision 63–4
  Wu Cheng-i 15, 22
  wu lun 97
  Yellow Emperor's Classic of Internal Medicine, The 8, 152
  Yellow Mountain criteria 146–7